A Problem-Solving Approach

HELPING CANCER PATIENTS COPE

Arthur M. Nezu · Christine Maguth Nezu

Stephanie H. Friedman · Shirley Faddis · Peter S. Houts

American Psychological Association

Washington, DC

Published by
American Psychological Association
750 First Street, NE
Washington, DC 20002

Copies may be ordered from
APA Order Department
P.O. Box 92984
Washington, DC 20090-2984

In the U.K., Europe, Africa, and the Middle East, copies may be ordered from
American Psychological Association
3 Henrietta Street
Covent Garden, London
WC2E 8LU England

Typeset in Meridien by Harlowe Typography, Cottage City, MD

Printer: Braun-Brumfield, Inc., Ann Arbor, MI
Cover Designer: Minker Design, Bethesda, MD
Technical/Production Editor: Catherine R. W. Hudson
Cover Photo: Corbis-Bettmann

Library of Congress Cataloging-in-Publication Data
Helping cancer patients cope : a problem-solving approach / Arthur M.
   Nezu ... [et al.].
       p. cm.
   Includes bibliographical references and index.
   ISBN 1-55798-533-2 (casebound : acid-free paper)
   1. Cancer—Psychological aspects. 2. Adjustment (Psychology)
I. Nezu, Arthur M.
   [DNLM: 1. Neoplasms—psychology. 2. Adaptation, Psychological.
3. Problem Solving. QZ 200H483 1998]
RC262.H44 1999
616.99'4'0019—dc21
DNLM/DLC   98-36683
for Library of Congress   CIP

British Library Cataloguing-in-Publication Data
A CIP record is available from the British Library.

Printed in the United States of America
First Edition

This book is dedicated to the millions
of cancer patients and their families
who display extraordinary courage each day.

Contents

IV
ADAPTATION OF PROBLEM-SOLVING THERAPY FOR CAREGIVER TRAINING

Exhibits

Acknowledgments

This book and Project Genesis, the research protocol on which it is based, was supported by a grant from the National Cancer Institute (R01-CA61313) awarded to Arthur M. Nezu, PhD, principal investigator. We wish also to extend our sincere thanks to the multitude of physicians, social workers, and nursing staff who supported our research and clinical efforts, as well as the large number of problem-solving therapists, clinical assessors, and research assistants who worked diligently on behalf of this project.

THE NATURE OF CANCER AND COPING

Cancer and Its Consequences

1

Like most wars, the "war on cancer" leaves casualties, scars, and lives in need of healing in its wake. This book is a direct outgrowth of Project Genesis, a clinical research program funded by the National Cancer Institute. Project Genesis was developed to help adult cancer patients heal their lives through a problem-solving-based psychosocial intervention. During the past two decades, problem-solving training has increasingly been applied as a means of helping to improve the quality of life for individuals experiencing a wide range of chronic and acute difficulties (D'Zurilla & Nezu, in press). For example, over 10 years ago, we formulated a problem-solving model of major depression, which led to the development of a highly effective treatment modality for this affective disorder (A. M. Nezu, Nezu, & Perri, 1989). More recently, we have turned our research and clinical attention to the psychosocial needs of cancer patients (A. M. Nezu, Nezu, Friedman, Houts, & Faddis, 1997).

Problem-solving therapy (PST) represents a coping-skills training approach, whereby the individual (or couple, family, or group) is taught to use a series of tasks or operations geared to resolve complex and stressful problems. Its ultimate goal is to help improve people's coping ability, which can lead to a decrease in emotional distress, as well as to an improvement in their overall quality of life. As one Genesis patient put it, "Thanks to the problem-solving program, I was able to face my fear of a cancer recurrence and now have the tools to be very positive and confident about handling such a possibility."

It has only been recently that the community of health and mental health professionals has focused on the psychosocial needs of cancer patients and their families. An increasing awareness of the significant emotional, interpersonal, family, vocational, and functional problems experienced by such individuals, and how these problems potentially affect their health, quality of life, and even health outcome, have led to the creation of the field of *psychosocial oncology* or *psychooncology*. According to Holland (1990), the two major areas of interest characterizing this cancer subspecialty involve the following: "(a) the impact of cancer on the psychological function of the patient, the patient's family, and staff; and (b) the role that psychological and behavioral variables may have in cancer risk and survival" (p. 11). Embedded in these areas are questions concerning the potential efficacy of psychosocial interventions to improve a cancer patient's quality of life. It is for this purpose that we developed Project Genesis.

The present volume, in essence, represents a detailed treatment manual for conducting PST for adult cancer patients. In Section I, we describe the profound and extensive psychosocial difficulties that cancer patients often experience. In addition, we present the theory underlying this particular form of psychosocial treatment, the research base supporting its general efficacy, and the rationale for its particular applicability for the experience of cancer patients. Section II provides an overview of PST for cancer patients, including the process of the therapy; the related clinical issues; and the goals of the first, introductory, session. Section III contains a detailed treatment guide to conduct PST for cancer patients, including a series of patient handouts, "homework assignments," and sample exercises. To illustrate various therapeutic strategies and training modules, we describe two cases that are followed throughout the training. Finally, in Section IV, we provide a chapter that describes our problem-solving principles that have been adapted to caregiver education.

Before we describe PST, we present a brief overview of cancer and its psychosocial consequences.

Cancer Overview

WHAT IS CANCER?

Although many people think of cancer as being a single disease, it is in fact a term used to describe over 200 different diseases. However, all types of cancer have one characteristic in common—the uncontrollable growth and accumulation of abnormal cells. Normal cells behave according to a preprogrammed genetic set of rules unique to a particular cell type (e.g., skin, blood, and brain). They divide, mature, die, and are replaced according to this orderly plan. Cancer cells, on the other hand, do not follow biological rules—they divide more rapidly than usual, grow in a disorderly fashion, and do not properly mature.

Immortal cells are those cancer cells that do not know when to stop dividing or when to die. They can destroy normal surrounding tissue and tend to spread throughout the body. This abnormal process of *malignancy* leads to the accumulation of cancer cells that eventually form a mass or a *tumor*. If the proliferation of this cancerous growth is not stopped, the abnormal cells can extend to surrounding areas and *metastasize* or spread to form tumors in other parts of the body. Eventually, the affected organs and body systems cannot perform their functions, which may lead to death.

CANCER STATISTICS

During 1997, it was estimated that close to 1.4 million new cases of invasive cancer were diagnosed in the United States (American Cancer Society, 1997). Since 1990, approximately 10 million new cancer cases have been diagnosed. More than 1,500 people are expected to die each day from cancer this year. Cancer is the second leading cause of death in the United States, surpassed only by heart disease—one out of every four deaths in the United States is cancer related. Table 1 provides a breakdown of the estimated incidence of new cases by major cancer type (American Cancer Society, 1997).

Gender

At every age, men are found to be at a higher risk for cancer than women. Rates for 1997 indicate an overall estimate of 785,000 new cases for men and 596,000 new cases for women (American Cancer Society, 1997). Prostate cancer is the most common form of this disease in men, whereas breast cancer is the leading malignancy in women.

Race

The incidence of cancer varies widely among various ethnic groups in the United States (American Cancer Society, 1997). Among men, cancer rates are highest among African Americans, followed by Whites. Cancer rates among American Indian and Asian American men tend

---

TABLE 1

Major cancer types, estimated new cases, and known risk factors

Cancer type	New cases	Risk factors
Breast	180,200[a]	Family history of breast cancer, early menarche, late menopause, lengthy exposure to postmenopausal estrogens, recent use of oral contraceptives, no children, first birth at a late age, and higher education and SES
Cervix	14,500	First intercourse at early age, multiple sex partners, cigarette smoking, and low SES
Colon/Rectum	131,200	Family history of colorectal cancer or polyps, inflammatory bowel disease, physical inactivity, and inadequate intake of fruits and vegetables
Endometrium	34,900	Estrogen-related exposures (e.g., tamoxifen, early menarche, estrogen replacement therapy, never having children, diabetes, gallbladder disease, hypertension, and obesity)
Leukemia	28,300	Causes are generally unknown; Down's syndrome and other genetic abnormalities have higher incidence than usual
Lung	178,100	Cigarette smoking, exposure to certain industrial substances (e.g., arsenic, asbestos, and radon), radiation exposure, air pollution, and tuberculosis
Lymphoma	61,100	Largely unknown; reduced immune function may be risk factor
Oral cavity/Pharynx	30,750	Cigarette, pipe, cigar smoking; smokeless tobacco; and excessive alcohol consumption
Ovary	26,800	Age, never having children, family history of breast cancer or ovarian cancer, and breast cancer
Pancreas	27,600	Little is known; smoking
Prostate	334,500	Age, race (African Americans have highest incidence rate in the world)
Skin	900,000	Excessive exposure to ultraviolet radiation, fair complexion, and occupational exposure (e.g., coal tar, arsenic, and radium), family history, and atypical nevi (i.e., moles)
Urinary bladder	54,500	Smoking and exposure to dye, rubber, leather in urban areas

Note. Data from the American Cancer Society (1997). SES = Socioeconomic status.
[a]Indicates number of women.

to be low. Among women, differences as a function of race are less pronounced. It is possible that socioeconomic status has more to do with these differences than genetic background. For example, poverty, poor eating habits, limited access to care, and decreased knowledge base can all contribute to increased cancer incidence.

Improvement in Survival Rates

Approximately 7.4 million Americans who have a history of cancer are alive today (American Cancer Society, 1997). Some of these individuals are considered to be "cured," whereas the others continue to show evidence of cancer. Although there has been an increase in the mortality rates in the United States during the second half of the twentieth century, this has largely been due to the increase in lung cancer. When deaths attributed to this cancer type are excluded, cancer mortality actually shows a decrease of approximately 16% since 1950.

More important as an indicator that there is significant progress in the war on cancer is the improvement in survival rates. Early in this century, few patients diagnosed with cancer were expected to live. In the 1930s, the survival rate was about 1 in 4. This 5-year survival rate has improved during the past 60 years—approximately 4 in 10 cancer patients are expected to be alive 5 years after they are diagnosed (American Cancer Society, 1997). The metric of a 5-year survival rate is the commonly used benchmark to evaluate progress.

Risk Factors

Risk factors (see Table 1) concerning the development of cancer fall into several categories. First, genetic disposition, as represented by a positive family history of cancer, can play a role. For example, daughters of women who have breast cancer have a higher propensity to develop cancer of the breast than women who have no family history. Children who develop neuroblastoma or Wilms' tumor also have a genetic disposition to cancer development.

Second, exposure to certain viruses can lead to cancer development. For example, chronic hepatitis has been linked to liver cancer, whereas papilloma virus has been associated with cervical cancer. In addition, human immunodeficiency virus (HIV) has been associated with an increased risk of Hodgkin's lymphoma, B-cell lymphoma, and Kaposi's sarcoma.

Third, iatrogenic risks involving certain drugs, such as estrogen therapy and antineoplastics (e.g., alkylating agents), especially cyclophosphamide and busulfan, have also been found to be a risk factor.

Lifestyle factors, such as tobacco use, alcohol use, dietary intake, and sexual practices, entail a fourth category of cancer risk variables. Tobacco use is responsible for nearly one in five deaths in the United States. It is strongly associated with lung, oral, esophagus, and bladder cancer. About one third of the cancer deaths in America are due to dietary factors. For example, increased dietary intake of fat is associated with breast and prostate cancer. Early sexual activity with many partners also increases the risk of cancer development.

Finally, occupational and environmental risk factors include chemical exposure, ultraviolet light, radon, and passive smoking exposure. The risk of lung cancer is enhanced by chemicals such as vinyl chloride and asbestos fibers. Ultraviolet light exposure over time increases the risk for skin cancer, as does the genetic predisposition to light or fair skin.

Cancer Classification Systems

TUMOR GRADES

Tumors are classified in terms of their differentiation. Tumor cells are said to be *differentiated* if they closely resemble their normal, healthy counterparts. Cancer cells that are dissimilar are called *undifferentiated* or *anaplastic*. The degree of cell differentiation plays an important role in making treatment decisions. High-grade tumors are generally fast growing, aggressive, and undifferentiated. Oncologists generally use four classifications to describe tumor grades: Grade I (70–100% differentiated), Grade II (50–75% differentiated), Grade III (25–50% differentiated), and Grade IV (under 25% differentiated).

STAGING

Cancers are also classified according to *stages* as a means of determining how far a cancer has progressed and according to whether and where it has spread. Labeled *0* to *IV*, there are five cancer stages. In addition, depending on the type of cancer, stages are sometimes subdivided (e.g., IIA and IIB). The higher the stage, the more advanced the cancer. Practically, a cancer in the early stage will likely be small and confined to a primary site. Advanced-stage cancers will likely be large and have spread to lymph nodes or other structures.

TNM SYSTEM

The American Joint Commission on Cancer developed another means of classifying cancers and incorporated three cancer variables: *T* (tumor), *N* (nodes), and *M* (metastasis). The T relates to the size of the primary tumor and whether it has invaded nearby tissues and structures. The N involves the degree to which lymph nodes have been affected by the primary tumor. M refers to whether the cancer has spread to other organs and the degree to which it has metastasized.

Cancer Treatment

Cancer treatment generally falls into four major categories: surgery, radiation, chemotherapy, and biological therapy. Any of these approaches can be used as a *primary* treatment, which is the major intervention for a particular cancer type. *Adjuvant therapy* is given after the primary treatment has been implemented as part of a comprehensive treatment protocol. For example, a woman may have surgery to remove a breast tumor (primary treatment), which may be followed by chemotherapy (adjuvant therapy). Adjuvant therapy helps to eliminate those microscopic cancer cells that are not possible to remove during surgery. *Neo-adjuvant therapy* occurs prior to the primary treatment in order to control known or potential sites of metastasis. *Prophylactic treatment* is targeted to a site where there is a high risk for cancer development. Small-cell carcinoma of the lung, for example, has a high propensity for metastasis to the brain. Prophylactic radiation therapy is given to the brain to prevent metastasis.

Most cancer types are treated with a multimodal approach. However, small local tumors with no possibility of metastasis can be treated with a single-modality intervention approach. Small, early skin cancers and early colon cancer are examples of tumors in which single-modality treatment is appropriate. Some leukemias are treated only with chemotherapy. However, multimodal treatment is more common and is the standard for large, bulky tumors and tumors with a propensity to spread. For example, breast, lung, and gynecological cancers are usually treated with multiple modalities.

The goals of cancer therapy fall into three categories: cure, control, and palliation. *Cure* is achievable for some tumors, such as testicular, cervical, and skin cancer. The maximal risk of disease recurrence usually occurs within the first 2 years after a primary treatment. Therapy aimed at *control* is used for tumors for which there is no possible cure. Control is defined as containment of the tumor. *Palliation* is aimed at the comfort and relief of symptoms when cure is impossible. This treatment goal may use the same therapeutic agents; however, a shorter course is given.

SURGERY

Surgery is the oldest form of cancer treatment. More cancers are cured with surgery than any other treatment form. In addition to cure, surgery has many roles. Benign tumors that are precancerous are removed with various surgical procedures. This is considered *prophylactic surgery*. For example, a woman who has had breast cancer may have her second breast removed to reduce the risk of cancer recurrence. Removal of a primary tumor is a major use of surgery. Major surgery involves removing the tumor, surrounding tissue, and lymph nodes. Major surgery is also performed to remove other tumors that are metastatic, recurrent, or residual. Palliative surgery improves quality of life by relieving obstructive symptoms.

Reconstruction is useful for those individuals who have had a major surgery to remove a tumor that has deformed or caused a functional problem. Breast reconstruction is a common example. Depending on the tumor's location in the breast, mastectomies remain the most logical surgery choice. Reconstruction can occur at the time of surgery or after a period of healing has occurred.

Finally, surgery is used to support other treatment modalities, such as chemotherapy or radiation. Surgeons insert various types of catheters and implantable devices that allow efficient delivery of chemotherapeutic agents. Devices can be surgically placed in the venous system, a major organ (e.g., gastrotomy tubes into the stomach), the brain (e.g., ventricules), and cavities, such as the vaginal vault (e.g., radiation implants). Small pumps can be implanted to deliver chemotherapy directly into various organs, such as the liver, to maximize the effects of the therapy.

CHEMOTHERAPY

Chemotherapy is used for the treatment of hematological tumors and for solid tumors that have metastasized to another area. Chemotherapy can be used to cure, control, or palliate a cancerous process. Some malignancies, such as Hodgkin's disease and testicular cancer, can be cured by using chemotherapy as a single treatment. Tumors—such as breast, chronic lymphocytic leukemia, acute myelocytic leukemia, and soft tissue sarcomas—can be controlled with the use of chemotherapy. When the treatment goal is palliation, chemotherapy is used to reduce the tumor to relieve pressure on structures that are causing discomfort.

Chemotherapy acts by altering the cancer-cell life processes and functioning in various ways. Antineoplastic drug agents are classified by the specific actions each one has on the cell cycle process and biochemical structure. Because cells are constantly dividing and are in various phases of the cell cycle, several antineoplastic agents are used to provide the maximum "cell kill" possible without increasing the drug's toxicity.

Chemotherapy is a systemic intervention. The drug agents do not have the ability to select only the malignant cells, therefore, both normal and malignant cells are damaged by the antineoplastic agents. Side effects occur from the damage to rapidly dividing cells. Some agents damage other cells, such as renal cells, because of the agents' biochemical effects. For example, antineoplastic agents that are classified as vinca alkaloids are neurotoxic and can produce permanent neurologic damage. The most common side effects of chemotherapy include hair loss, low white-cell count, low platelet count, nausea, vomiting, diarrhea, and sore mouth. Because it is possible to develop a fatal infection or episode of extensive bleeding that is due to low white-cell and platelet count, patients must have regular blood counts while receiving chemotherapy. If the count indicates that the risk is high for an infection or bleeding episode, the treatment may be postponed until the count rises. The rest period is usually not long enough to allow time for the tumor to continue to grow or to spread uncontrolled. To minimize the chance of developing a serious infection, patients may be given colony-stimulating factors (CSFs) to boost the production of white cells. Side effects, such as hair loss, are temporary, and regrowth will begin after the treatment is discontinued.

RADIATION

Radiation therapy is also used to cure, control, and palliate various tumors. Tumors such as Hodgkin's disease, malignant skin tumors, cervical, and early-stage testicular cancers are curable today with the use of radiation therapy. Both bladder and late-stage breast cancer are controlled by using radiation. For many patients, the use of radiation assists in palliation of uncontrolled pain, metastatic brain tumors, and distressing obstructive symptoms resulting from superior vena cava syndrome or spinal cord compression.

Radiation works on the cellular level by using high-energy waves or particles. The cancer cells die because of the damaging effects of radiation on the cells' DNA molecules. The cellular DNA damage results in their eventual death. Normal cells within the field of treatment are also killed by radiation therapy, which can lead to side effects usually associated with radiation. However, normal cells have the capacity to repair themselves, whereas the cancer cells do not.

The side effects of radiation, unlike chemotherapy, are accumulative. Acute effects occur within the first 6 months of treatment.

Chronic effects occur after the first 6 months. Radiation affects both normal and cancerous cells that are rapidly growing. Normal rapidly dividing cells include skin, mucous membrane, hair follicles, bone marrow, and germ cells. Nausea, vomiting, diarrhea, hair loss, and anemia can result from radiation therapy, depending on the site location of the treatment. These side effects will resolve in time after the cells have had time to repair and to resume normal functioning. The most common side effect of radiation therapy is fatigue. Long-term effects of radiation therapy are usually the result of permanent cell damage in the area receiving the therapy. Examples of chronic side effects are pulmonary pneumonitis, fibrosis (pulmonary and bladder), and sterility.

IMMUNOTHERAPY

The use of biological response modifiers (BRMs) to treat cancer is a newer treatment modality that uses the individual's own immune system to fight the tumor cells in order to engender a therapeutic response. BRMs are used for particular tumors such as hairy cell leukemia, melanoma, and renal cell carcinoma. The use of this modality is somewhat problematic in that the immune system does not always treat cancer cells as foreign. Cancer cells have the ability to alter the cell membrane such that the immune system does not "read" it as abnormal. The three most commonly known BRMs are interferon (INF), interleukin-2 (IL-2), and CSFs. These are highly purified proteins that are administered to activate, modify, enhance, or restore the immune system. There is a group of BRMs that exhibits some antitumor effects that remain investigational at this time. The CSFs are used to treat the reduced white cell count associated with chemotherapy.

BRMs are natural body proteins and can be attached to radioisotopes and antineoplastic agents. They are administered orally, subcutaneously, intravenously, intraperitoneally, intraarterially, and intracavitarily. Although these agents are natural proteins found in the body, when they are administered therapeutically, they can produce uncomfortable side effects. The most common is a flulike syndrome consisting of headaches, fever, chills, and muscle and joint aches and pains. In addition, certain BRMs (e.g., high-dose IL-2) can cause capillary leak syndrome, which is a potentially life-threatening situation. This is characterized by fluid leaking from the capillaries into interstitial spaces, resulting in reduced blood pressure, rapid weight gain, and respiratory distress. If not corrected, capillary leak syndrome can result in kidney failure and possible death from respiratory arrest.

BONE MARROW TRANSPLANTATION

During the 1970s and 1980s, advancements in laboratory techniques have made bone marrow transplantation (BMT) a viable treatment option for a select group of patients. For some disease entities, a BMT can extend life or even cure a hematologic malignancy. However, for many solid tumors, BMT remains experimental and is not considered an option. The diagnoses for which a BMT may be a treatment option include aplastic anemia, leukemias, lymphomas, Hodgkin's disease, breast cancer, and multiple myeloma.

Bone marrow is located in the iliac crest, sternum, long bones, and ribs. The marrow contains the blood-forming components that manufacture red cells, white cells, and platelets. In the marrow and circulating blood (peripheral), an immature cell, called a *stem cell*, exists that is the "parent" cell for the development of red cells, white cells, and platelets. If the marrow becomes malignant (i.e., leukemia), the blood-forming process is altered and results in a life-threatening situation. The individual then becomes at risk for lethal infections or hemorrhaging. If the marrow can be destroyed and replaced with normal marrow free from the malignant cells, the malignancy can potentially be cured.

There are several types of BMTs. An *autologous* transplant is one in which the recipient donates the marrow for infusion at a later time. A *syngeneic* transplant is performed when the recipient has a genetically identical twin. *Allogeneic* transplants require a marrow donation from a related or unrelated donor. For a recipient to receive an allogeneic transplant, histocompatibility testing must be performed to obtain the closest possible genetic match. Allogeneic transplant recipients are at risk for developing graft-versus-host (GVH) disease, which can potentially be lethal.

After a BMT, the patient is supported with antibiotics, immune-suppressing agents, and nutritional supplements. The period of pancytopenia (i.e., low blood count) lasts between 10 and 30 days. Engraftment of the marrow can be expected around the 14th day after the transplant. Patients who have received an allogeneic transplant are at risk for GVH disease, which is the result of the new marrow rejecting the recipient.

Because a detailed description of the pathophysiology, means of diagnosis, and medical complications of cancer is far beyond the scope of this book, at the end of this chapter, we provide a list of recommended readings that can also be offered to cancer patients themselves as valuable sources of information. We strongly encourage the mental health professional to be familiar with this material in order to best communicate with the cancer patient about his or her condition.

In the next section, we focus on the psychosocial sequella of cancer and its treatment.

Psychosocial Consequences of Cancer

Considerable progress has been made in effectively treating cancer. Statistically speaking, the answer to the question, "Will I die?" in response to hearing the diagnosis of cancer is no. Many forms are curable, and there is a sustained decline in the overall death rate from cancer when one focuses on the impact on the total population (Murphy, Morris, & Lange, 1997). Because of improvements in medical science, however, more people are living with cancer than ever before. Although the extensive medical needs of such patients may be well attended to, psychosocial and emotional needs are often overlooked (Houts, Yasko, Kahn, Schelzel, & Marconi, 1986). Almost every aspect of one's life can be overturned, as cancer engenders many stressors and can lead to significantly compromised quality of life. Even for people who historically have coped well with major negative life events, cancer and its treatment greatly increase the stressful nature of even routine daily tasks. Weisman and Worden (1976–1977) referred to this situation for cancer patients as an "existential plight," in which one's very existence may be endangered. Recognizably, not every individual diagnosed with cancer will experience a plethora of problems, but most patients do report significant difficulties. These problems can be intrapersonal, social, or environmental in nature.

INTRAPERSONAL DIFFICULTIES

Experiencing cancer requires substantial adaptation to change. For example, biological changes related to physical appearance, hormonal activity, and general health can require significant psychosocial adjustment. These changes can negatively affect sexual functioning, psychological health, and overall well-being. Changes in behavior may be required during treatment and recovery from cancer. For example, patients may be required to decrease or discontinue specific behaviors, such as smoking or alcohol use. Patients' diets, eating patterns, and exercise regimens may need to be altered. Medical staff may prescribe various behavioral changes to improve the efficacy of treatment protocols and to reduce the risk of negative effects of treatment. For instance, personal and dental hygiene must be attended to with increased care; adherence to medical prescriptions may dictate scrupulous record keeping.

Cancer can also affect one's view of life. For example, Weisman and Worden (1976–1977) found that persons with cancer who experienced high levels of emotional distress were found to be pessimistic, tending to give up easily and to expect little support. Such individuals also reported having more interpersonal and intrapersonal difficulties prior to their diagnosis of cancer. During the course of treatment, they perceived more health concerns, doubts about treatment, and a worse prognosis.

Emotionally, the most common types of psychological disturbance evidenced in cancer patients are depression and anxiety. Although such emotional distress is a normal outcome of cancer and its treatment, many patients experience levels that are clinically significant (Meyerowitz, 1983). Estimates of the prevalence of significant psychological difficulties range between 23% and 66% of studied cancer patient populations (Telch & Telch, 1986). With regard to depression, for example, Massie and Holland (1988) found that the most common reason for psychiatric consultations among a sample of 546 cancer patients was depression, suicide risk, or both. Major depression was observed in 20% of this sample, and adjustment disorder with depressed mood in another 27%. Other studies have found the prevalence rate of depression among cancer patients to be as high as 58% (Hinton, 1972) and 56% (Levine, Silberfarb, & Lipowski, 1978). Only a small number of cancer patients are found to have a preexisting affective disorder (< 6%; Locke & Regier, 1985), underscoring the causal role of cancer regarding depression.

By far the most common form of anxiety among cancer patients is reactive in nature—it can be produced by the diagnosis, pain, underlying medical condition, medication side effects, and related psychosocial problems. In Hinton's (1972) study of 50 terminally ill cancer patients, 42% were found to be anxious. Sixty-two of 546 psychiatric consultations involved a diagnosis of adjustment-disorder anxious type in the study by Massie and Holland (1988), whereas 22 involved actual anxiety disorders. Other types of anxiety reactions include phobias, posttraumatic stress disorder, and anticipatory nausea. Similar to findings regarding depression among cancer patients, only 8% of such individuals are thought to have preexisting anxiety disorders (Massie, 1990).

Reports about the incidence of suicide vary greatly (Breitbart, 1990), ranging from estimates suggesting that it is similar to that of the general population (Fox, Stanek, Boyd, & Flannery, 1982) to estimates indicating that it is 2–10 times greater (e.g., Whitlock, 1978). The actual incidence is probably underestimated because of the reluctance by family members to report death by suicide (Holland, 1982). There is some evidence to suggest that suicide is more prevalent among patients with oral, pharyngeal, and lung cancers (e.g., Bolund, 1985). As depression and hopelessness are often causally linked to suicide (Beck, Kovacs, & Weissman, 1975), the degree to which cancer patients experience these feelings increases their vulnerability to suicide as one option to deal with cancer.

Cancer and its treatment are associated with additional problems. For example, with far-advanced cancers across all types, approximately 70% of cancer patients have significant pain sometime during the course of treatment (Foley & Sundaresen, 1985). Unfortunately, some researchers have estimated that about 25% of cancer patients die without adequate relief from pain (Twycross & Lack, 1983). Other problems include sexual dysfunctions, fatigue, hair loss, loneliness, and appetite difficulties (Houts, Nezu, Nezu, Bucher, & Lipton, 1994).

INTERPERSONAL PROBLEMS

Interpersonal problems may span across a wide range of people (e.g., spouse–partner, family, children, and friends) and situations (e.g., career, job, education, religion, finances, sex, physical health, leisure, and personal goal attainment). Many cancer patients are unable to work for at least a limited time during the course of their treatment or recovery. Meeting some of the demands of the physical environment, as well as daily tasks and responsibilities, may require dependence on others. Added burdens on family or friends, in turn, may challenge already tenuous relationships. For example, costs of medical care and medications may exceed available financial resources, which may, in turn, exacerbate marital difficulties. In addition, parents with small children may not be able to provide adequate care for their family.

Cancer still maintains the stigma of a "death sentence" or that it could be contagious in some way (Garcia & Lee, 1989). These fallacies, though less prevalent than 20 years ago, create additional complications for persons in treatment for the disease and their families. For instance, people may feel ashamed or embarrassed by their diagnosis, which may cause them to alienate themselves from others. Given that the literature suggests many positive effects that result from perceived social support (Rowland, 1990a, 1990b), isolation or alienation can be particularly troublesome. In addition, many people do not know how to respond to family members of cancer patients and, therefore, say nothing at all. Others may avoid persons with cancer because of apparent baldness, weight loss, or sickness.

From another perspective, the social environment can present problems to persons with cancer who have ambulatory limitations that are due to fatigue, muscle weakness, neuropathy, or amputation. Furthermore, persons whose immune systems are compromised because of treatment will be restricted regarding active participation in social activities as well. Because cancer patients are at a higher risk for infection, they may be restricted from many enclosed public places where germs flourish, such as restaurants or movie theaters. Similarly, persons with cancer may have less opportunity to meet new people or to participate in social events during the time of treatment and recovery.

PROBLEMS IN THE PHYSICAL ENVIRONMENT

Some of the obstacles that are commonly experienced include meeting instrumental physical needs, such as arranging transportation for medical appointments, executing activities of daily living (e.g., bathing or dressing oneself), preparing meals, or simply walking to the bathroom or second floor in one's own home. Independent living may be compromised during treatment. Numerous other complications may arise from the physical and logistical aspects of a cancer diagnosis and treatment, independent of non-cancer-related stressors.

Pathway of Patients' Psychosocial Experiences

To highlight some of the specific obstacles and problems that individuals with cancer may face during the course of their diagnosis and treatment, in this next section, we provide an overview of the psychosocial "clinical pathway" that patients may undergo. Although the majority of what is described emphasizes the negative aspects and strains of a cancer diagnosis, it is important to note that many individuals report positive outcomes of their diagnosis. For example, some patients find positive meaning in their illness, become closer to family members or friends, find new strengths within themselves, or restore or find faith in their religion. Yet even these individuals are not free of the complexities introduced by cancer. Each step of the diagnosis and treatment process presents new problems or difficulties for which patients may commonly seek psychological treatment.

THE DIAGNOSIS

Often cancer is diagnosed in response to a patient's complaints of fatigue, weakness, excessive coughing, or other flulike symptoms. Or perhaps, persons feel isolated pain that they thought to be a muscle strain. Others may have had cancer detected without the presence of symptoms, such as during yearly physical exams or dental appointments. Thus, most people recall the instant that they learned of their diagnosis as "shocking," "frightening," or even "surreal." Some individuals have difficulty recalling the actual meeting with their physicians because of the intensity of disbelief or the fear instilled by the words "you have cancer." For this reason, many physicians prefer that this information be given to the patient in the presence of a family member or significant other. The conversation that immediately follows the devastating news does not always "register" with the cancer patient, who, from that moment forward, is consumed by his or her preconception of what a diagnosis of cancer means.

Initially, people newly diagnosed with cancer may deny that they have a life-threatening chronic illness. Others may accept the diagnosis of cancer but may deny the implications of the disease. Depending on a person's preexisting coping style, the denial may be an acute reaction to the unexpected information, or it may be a more pervasive coping response. For some, the denial may be so significant that treatment is delayed beyond medical recommendations, which can have fatal consequences (Kunkel, Woods, Rodgers, & Myers, 1997).

Patients often seek to explain how or why they came to develop cancer. This question may remain unanswered in their minds for an unspecified duration. Attributional styles, religious beliefs, cultural traditions, and many other factors may contribute to the explanation that persons adopt. Once patients accept the reality of their medical status, it is normal for them to experience anger. Anger may be externalized or directed toward others. Persons with cancer may be angry at their medical team for not detecting the cancer sooner. They may be angry that technology has not discovered a cure for their disease. People who have been exposed to environmental hazards because of their jobs may be angry with their employer for not taking more precautions. They may be angry at family members who did not serve as better role models to engage in health-promoting behaviors. People who have not lived religious or "pure lives" may feel angry at their "Divine Superior," or they may feel that they are being punished.

Persons who have a more internalized locus of control may lament in anger toward themselves or have guilty feelings regarding their diagnosis. Patients may express guilt for not having lived a healthier life by maintaining better eating habits or engaging in more exercise. People who smoke or consume excessive amounts of alcohol may also feel guilty or ashamed because they believe that they brought the cancer upon themselves. If persons have a medical history of cancer in their family, they may feel guilty for not engaging in self-examinations or medical screenings. Conversely, persons who consider themselves to be healthy individuals because they have taken good care of themselves may have a particularly hard time attributing their diagnosis to any specific causal factor. This uncertainty can be equally, if not more, disconcerting.

Beyond anger and guilt, cancer patients typically experience a combination of other emotions once their "plight" has become a reality to them. It is common for people to report depressed feelings, fear of treatment, fear of dying, and the uncertainty that often cannot be immediately demystified regarding their future. Many patients also report feeling isolated by their diagnosis. They may believe that close friends and family are trying to comfort them. However, many cancer patients do not believe that others can truly understand how they feel unless they have had a diagnosis of cancer themselves. Others may isolate themselves by keeping their diagnosis confidential. They may choose not to disclose their medical status because they are afraid of others' reactions; they do not want to be perceived as "sickly" or different.

Although the emotional aspects of the disease are understandable, the progressive nature of the disease may not allow for persons to have an extensive time period to contemplate their situation. Persons with cancer are immediately forced to think about their financial status, advanced directives or living wills, and treatment options, among other psychosocial issues. If they are the first person within their family to have cancer, they may have little knowledge about what to expect during the course of their disease. Seeking treatment options may require sophisticated self-education regarding clinical trials, specialists, comprehensive treatment centers, location and travel to treatment, and other logistical concerns. Again, depending on their premorbid coping style, individuals may seek a tremendous amount of information regarding the diagnosis, or they may choose to learn only the minimal amount of information necessary to consent to treatment. Regardless, even the most basic amount of information that is required to be disclosed is likely to be incredibly overwhelming. This may be an ideal time to introduce coping-skills training to help people learn more effective ways to deal with their emotional reactions. Learning new ways to cope would help to prevent emotions from interfering with rational decision making regarding treatment and planning for the near and distant future.

BECOMING A "PATIENT"

Treatment for cancer is often described as "worse than the disease itself." This is especially true for patients who experienced no symptoms of their cancer when it was detected. As described earlier, patients typically receive chemotherapy, radiation, surgery, biological therapy, or a combination of these interventions.

More than 50 types of drugs are used in chemotherapy treatment, therefore, the side effects experienced may vary greatly. Some people lose their hair as a result of chemotherapy. Many patients experience nausea and vomiting. Persons receiving high-dose chemotherapy may suffer from mouth sores that have been likened to "craters." Diarrhea can also occur when chemotherapy drugs affect the lining of the intestines.

Fatigue is the most common side effect of radiation treatment, regardless of the site of the cancer. The radiation "burns" and temporary change in skin pigmentation are common sources of distress for persons receiving this type of treatment. Other side effects of radiation therapy are specific to the location of the disease. For example, radiation to the throat is likely to cause soreness and difficulty in swallowing after several treatments. Many people receiving radiation lose their appetite.

Surgery may result in scarring or tenderness at the site of the operation. Soreness is common for at least a period of time during recovery. Body-image concerns may be heightened because of changes in appearance, the need for a prosthetic device, or an ostomy. Furthermore, patients sometimes have difficulty understanding why they must receive chemotherapy or radiation following surgery.

When persons with cancer begin their medical treatment, feelings of loss of control may increase. It may seem that the cancer is now in control and that they should feel well enough to engage in certain social or work-related activities. The cancer treatment regimens may dictate when patients have to be admitted into the hospital or may require frequent visits to an outpatient clinic. In the hospital, daily routines are based on hospital staff's schedules for meal service, showers, medical rounds, monitoring of vital signs, or medication distribution.

After discharge from the hospital, patients may initially be required to schedule frequent follow-up appointments with their oncologists. Chemotherapy or radiation therapy may be administered in an outpatient setting. Regardless, the constant waiting involved in most medical offices is another source of anxiety for persons anticipating test results, medical procedures, or consultation. At times, anxiety or fear of doctor appointments may lead to avoidance. When patients do attend their medical appointments, but experience an increase in anxiety, their treatment may seem worse, or they may not use it as an opportunity to ask questions of their medical team. Patients may become angry with their perceived loss of control in these settings as well.

During treatment and weakened physical states, family members or friends become instrumental in providing transportation to and from medical appointments. In addition, patients are often forced to rely on family members and friends to meet other basic needs, such as meal preparation or bedside care. For persons who have typically been in the caretaker role (e.g., caring for children or assuming household duties), being incapacitated and having to depend on others can exacerbate negative mood states, such as feelings of helplessness or guilt. Persons who are the primary generator of income may feel inadequate or worthless if they are not able to continue to work. Moreover, if intimacy or sexual contact is compromised because of negative feelings or physical discomfort, persons may be concerned about their marital or partner relationships. When persons are compromised by cancer in their parental roles, the parents' well-being, as well as the children's well-being, may be at risk. Many parents seek guidance in helping their children cope when cancer strikes their family. Children may misbehave more frequently because of the lessened attention that they may receive from the ill family member. These behavioral changes are another common source of stress and negative feelings for many cancer patients.

Not everyone is fortunate to have family members or friends to rely on in times of crisis. Individuals without strong social support networks may be forced to be temporarily admitted to nursing homes or to hire home nursing care. It is also not uncommon for friends or family members to distance themselves from persons with cancer for a variety of reasons (i.e., not knowing what to say, fear of the disease, and not wanting to burden the patient with phone calls or visits). Patients may experience rejection or distress if coworkers, friends, or relatives do not attempt to be supportive. Conversely, friends or family members may make efforts to be supportive, yet, the patient may perceive their efforts as insufficient. For example, patients may respond negatively to others' behaviors that do not meet their expectations. Therefore, some patients may become upset if family or friends become overprotective, do not show enough interest, show too much interest, or treat the patient too much like a "patient" or not enough like a patient.

In addition to the changing roles within the family structure, other role changes may contribute to the difficulty in adjusting to a cancer diagnosis. During the course of medical treatment, whether it is surgery, radiation, chemotherapy, biological therapy, or a combination of these regimens, patients are likely to experience fatigue, weakness, and loss of energy. Depending on the site of surgery or radiation, patients may also experience localized pain or immobility. For individuals who are able to continue to work during treatment, scheduling medical appointments with minimal interference with work schedules may be challenging. Depending on a company's policy, persons may be required to use up sick leave or vacation time. Beyond this allowance, many patients are forced by financial needs to work part time. Others may take unpaid leaves of absence and possibly face financial hardship. If treatment requires extended absence, persons may be terminated from their position, creating additional stresses for the future. In some situations, cancer and its treatment may prevent persons from remaining within the same career path. For example, a person with cancer of the larynx will not be able to return to his or her job as a telemarketer, or a nurse who had an allogenic bone marrow transplant will not be permitted to be exposed to sick individuals for a minimum of 6 months to 1 year posttransplant.

ONGOING TREATMENT

Physicians will typically try to give patients an approximate time line of proposed treatment specific to their cancer diagnosis. Yet, for many people, the length of necessary treatment is not always clear and certainly cannot be guaranteed. Treatment regimens may be prescribed noncommitally until the cancer's response to the intervention can be evaluated. Some individuals will continue in treatment for the duration of their life, either for palliative care or for maintenance of their disease state. Thus, it is conceivable that some persons remain in the patient role indefinitely.

When treatment is limited, many gain comfort in knowing that they will resume some essence of "normality" in the near or distant future. However, persons who did not anticipate lengthy ongoing treatment may experience increased feelings of hopelessness, suicidality, depression, and a poor outlook on the future. It is likely that persons who receive continued treatment for their cancer will not have the same level of support from all friends and family members as they did at the time of the initial diagnosis. Furthermore, children have difficulty understanding why the parent is always sick. Even the most understanding employers have to evaluate the economic cost–benefit of frequent absences that are due to medical leave. Financial situations are unlikely to improve, and the cost of medical care continues to rise.

Individuals who are given the choice of continuing treatment as a prophylactic measure are faced with a unique situation. The difficulty of this decision is likely to challenge the most rational and effective decision maker. In some cases, such as many forms of leukemia, physicians can predict with certainty that the cancer will return. However, with many types of cancer, the outcome is much more ambiguous. Therefore, when treatment is considered optional because of inconclusive scientific research, it is not certain that the cancer would return if patients do not choose continued treatment. Furthermore, the patient cannot be guaranteed that the return of cancer can be prevented, even with prophylactic treatment.

The outside observer may automatically assume that they would opt for prophylactic treatment if there was a possibility that it could prevent a recurrence. However, for individuals who have undergone chemotherapy or radiation treatment, because of their physical side effects, the emotional aspects of treatment, and other existential consequences, the choice is far from simple. Thus, the negative options they must choose between—continuing in the patient role versus dealing with potential feelings of uncertainty or regret if they do not—pose a tremendous challenge to individuals' coping abilities. Having to make this decision may influence patients to seek psychological counseling. Physicians may request psychological consultation if patients are exhibiting heightened distress with regard to their treatment choice or if patients do not seem to evaluate their options realistically.

WHEN CANCER TREATMENT DOES NOT WORK

For most types of cancer, many options for treatment exist. If traditional treatments have not been successful, persons may inquire about investigational or experimental treatments known as *clinical trials*. The outcomes of clinical trials are uncertain and to some degree are unpredictable. Yet, some people will unquestioningly enroll in such a protocol that provides them with a glimmer of hope for recovery. For many, this decision is much more complicated. Persons must evaluate their willingness to remain a patient without convincing statistics that treatment will prolong their life. The decision-making process includes evaluating priorities, moral or religious beliefs, family values, financial situations, and quantity of life versus quality of life. Patients need to make personal decisions as to when they are willing to shift their focus from seeking recovery to enhancing the quality of the time that they have remaining.

Individuals who choose only palliative care may experience increased distress as they recognize the implications of their prognosis. Persons in this phase of their disease will go through the cycles of the grieving process while facing their own mortality and thinking about their death's impact on family and friends. Some patients who choose to discontinue searching for a cure may experience guilty feelings, such as "Have I really tried everything?" or "Should I have continued in treatment for the sake of my family?" Other symptoms of depression and anxiety are also likely to increase.

When cancer cannot be controlled or cured, a new set of stressors and decisions arises that may or may not have been considered previously:

"Who will care for persons with cancer during their remaining time?" "Will they reside in their home, a nursing home, or hospital?" "What will become of their family, pets, home, assets, medical bills?" "Do they want to have input into their obituary or how they would like to be remembered?" "Are there funeral or burial arrangements that they would like to make to reduce the burden on family members?" "If there are young children involved, what can they do to prepare them?" "What can they do to prepare for their children's future?" "How can they be of help to their spouse or other family members?"

This represents only a partial list of relevant, practical questions or decisions to be made. Yet, this list is likely to make even a healthy person begin to feel overwhelmed. However, learning effective coping skills allows persons with cancer who have little or no hope for recovery to recognize that they can still be in control of the remainder of their life and the consequences of their death.

People facing death often fear the actual dying process, although they may or may not readily discuss this fear. Others may fear losing control at the end of their life. Fear may prevent them from discussing these concerns with their physicians or others and may lead them to avoid this topic altogether. Ironically, when fear or anxiety about death results in denial or avoidance, persons often forgo their decision making over aspects of their death for which they could take control. For example, people sometimes avoid or choose not to prepare their advanced directives or living will. Advanced directives are prepared in a signed document that describes the details of a person's wishes for medical care in the event that he or she is in an irreversible condition and is not able to speak or communicate for him- or herself. Unfortunately, when advanced directives have not been prepared, persons may be intubated or hooked up to machines for oxygen and complete cardiovascular support against what may have been their unknown wishes. Furthermore, persons who do not designate a durable power of attorney, a trustee of their estate, or a guardian for their children may create undue confusion or difficulties for their families upon death.

At the other extreme, patients may experience passive suicidal ideation in an attempt to gain control of their imminent death. Specifically, it is not uncommon for individuals who fear suffering, or who have suffered during the course of their disease, to plan or consider suicide as a measure to relieve themselves of pain (Breitbart, 1990).

THE ROAD TO RECOVERY

Given the extensive complications of arranging and receiving medical treatments, it would seem that ending treatment would be an overwhelmingly positive situation. Although few would contest the relief accompanied with knowing that doctor visits may be less frequent and that the unpleasantries of chemotherapy or radiation are behind them, there are many concerns that often remain. After an ongoing battle against the cancer, some people may find it difficult to end an active fight against the disease.

If an increase in anxiety results, it may be manifested in many ways. Individuals who have been determined "cancer free" may increase their attention to nutrition, diet, and exercise. In the extreme, thoughts about diet and exercise may become constant. For others, the ongoing fear of recurrence may preoccupy their thoughts. Reentering work environments or resuming responsibilities in social circles or family may be anxiety provoking, if individuals have doubts about their recovery or others' perception of their illness. People with cancer often describe feeling self-conscious of others' awareness of this heightened vulnerability. Even when people begin to feel better physically, body-image concerns and fears of mortality often linger.

Some cancer patients describe themselves as having been exclusively focused on treatment. These people may experience the height of their emotional reaction to the cancer once the treatment is over. Yet, family members and friends may be less supportive posttreatment because it is in the past. In these circumstances, individuals who have had cancer often claim that only other survivors of cancer, or trained professionals, can truly understand their feelings.

Other posttreatment interpersonal difficulties may arise in marital relationships, work environments, or social relationships. Sometimes others impose certain expectations on them regarding their recovery period. A common complaint, for example, is that when individuals are no longer receiving treatment or looking "sick," others unrealistically expect them to immediately manage the same level of activity as prior to their diagnosis. Spouses, partners, or friends may be less understanding of patients' lack of sexual desire, decreased energy, or change of interest in previously enjoyed activities or recreation. In fact, cancer patients' interests may change regarding social activities, work-related or relationship goals, or personal goals. Many recovering cancer patients describe a new outlook on life or a change in their priorities.

LIVING AS A SURVIVOR

In addition to the challenges of reentering work or resuming roles and responsibilities, the psychological responses encountered during the initial posttreatment phase of recovery as previously described may continue to pose challenges to survivors' coping ability and psychological well-being for an extended period of time (Tross & Holland, 1990).

Individuals who are determined cancer free are often given an estimated time frame to surpass to be considered cured of their disease. Prognoses are based on statistics that compare patients' disease states with large numbers of people who have had similar diseases. However, other variables such as age, comorbid health problems, and other factors are considered when a prognosis is determined for individual patients. For many types of cancer, individuals who are symptom free for 5 years posttreatment are considered to be cured.

Aside from the return of the initial diagnosis of cancer, individuals may experience adverse effects of treatment many years past the "anniversary date." Such effects may include organ dysfunction or failure, infection, bone deterioration, cataracts, or even a secondary diagnosis of cancer. Certain types of cancer treatment are actually carcinogenic, thus, people may be at a higher risk for developing a secondary diagnosis of cancer in the future. For example, Byrd (1983) found that the incidence of developing a second malignancy 20 years after treatment is approximately 17%, about 20 times that of the general population.

Individuals who are cancer free may have difficulty accepting that they are survivors of cancer because of these known possibilities of adverse effects, recurrence, or new diagnosis. Others may be at risk for psychological morbidity if they focus entirely on their anniversary date and are thus completely unprepared for the possibility that they may face a new experience with cancer in their future. Prior to the anniversary date, persons may feel excessive vulnerability or fear. Understanding this precarious situation of survivorship highlights the ongoing challenge with which individuals who have completed cancer treatment must learn to cope.

Sexual dysfunctions are also not uncommon in individuals who have successfully been treated for cancer and may be the reason some clients initiate contact with mental health professionals. Difficulties may occur as a result of physical, biological, or psychological changes, or a combination of these factors. During cancer treatment, the extent to which couples engage in intimate or sexual behavior varies considerably. After treatment, however, survivors or their spouses–partners may believe that they should be ready to engage in intimate or sexual behavior. Yet, there are a variety of reasons why intimate contact may be delayed. If infertility resulted from treatment, individuals may be confronting their feelings, beliefs, values, and morals surrounding this issue for the first time as a survivor.

As discussed previously, body-image concerns, decreased self-esteem, and heightened feelings of vulnerability may continue to be problematic. Additional psychological factors, such as anxiety and depression, may contribute to patients' global lack of interest in sexual contact. For men, anxiety is the most common psychological reason for erectile disorders reported in this population. Anxiety may be related to fear of recurrence, fear of germ transmission, or belief that cancer has damaged sexual functioning in some way. Individuals who have been celibate for an extended period of time may be nervous that their sexual performance has decreased in comparison to precancer or pretreatment performance. If the survivor's decreased sexual desire is not global, but rather specific to the partner, relationship or communication problems may be the root of the problem. Furthermore, partners may be afraid of causing harm to the survivor if they perceive them as weakened or fragile.

Physical factors that may cause decreased sexual desire may include fatigue, pain, or weakness. Changes in hormone levels may result from cancer treatment that may affect sexual functioning. For example, estrogen deficiency may cause vaginal mucosa to become thin and dry, therefore causing women pain during intercourse. Female androgen deficiency syndrome can decrease sexual desire as well. For men, gonadal functioning may change because of damaged germ cells or altered hormonal production that results in infertility or sterility. There are a variety of other physical changes that cause sexual dysfunction that are due to the specific types of chemotherapy, radiation, surgery, opiate pain medications, antidepressant or antipsychotic medications, aggressiveness of treatment, as well as comorbid health problems. Specific to the location of solid tumors or type of cancer, the prevalence of sexual dysfunction varies.

Once patients are finished with treatment, they enter a new phase of their cancer experience. Even when fears of mortality subside and individuals are considered cancer free or later cured, survivors of cancer often view life differently and face cancer-related challenges regularly. Survivors often recognize intrapersonal differences that are due to emotional, affective, physical, behavioral, and perceptual changes. Their new world view and their cancer experience are likely to have an effect on interpersonal relationships and environmental situations. Cancer patients often describe a heightened awareness of their surroundings, their daily activities, and their interactions with others. When survivors begin to adjust to no longer being a patient, they may report confusion, fear, depression, or a desire to refocus their efforts and to improve their quality of life.

Summary

The psychosocial consequences of cancer and its treatment can be substantial. Research has indicated that although emotional distress is a normal impact of this medical disease, many cancer patients experience levels that are clinically significant and require some form of psychological intervention. To provide the reader with a more clinically relevant picture of the difficulties and problems that a cancer patient must face, we described the psychosocial pathways beginning at initial diagnosis through living as a survivor.

The field of psychosocial oncology is fairly new (Holland & Rowland, 1990), thus offering few empirically based psychosocial interventions that can be used as guidelines for meeting the psychosocial needs of cancer patients. It is to that end that we have adapted our model of problem-solving coping-skills training, previously found highly effective for a variety of mental health disorders, to the plight of cancer patients. In the next chapter, we provide an overview of problem-solving therapy with regard to its theoretical underpinnings, research support, and clinical applications.

Recommended Readings Regarding Cancer

Altman, R., & Sarg, M. J. (1992). *The cancer dictionary.* New York: Facts on File, Inc.

Dollinger, M., Rosenbaum, E. H., & Cable, G. (1994). *Everyone's guide to cancer therapy: How cancer is diagnosed, treated, and managed day to day* (2nd ed.). Kansas City, MO: Andrews & McMeel.

Murphy, G. P., Morris, L., & Lange, D. (1997). *Informed decisions: The complete book of cancer diagnosis, treatment, and recovery.* New York: Viking.

A Problem-Solving
Conceptualization of Coping:
Theory, Research, and
Relevance to Cancer

2

The basic notion underlying the relevance of problem-solving therapy for cancer patients essentially lies in the moderating role that problem-solving coping serves regarding the general stress–distress relationship (A. M. Nezu & D'Zurilla, 1989; A. M. Nezu et al., 1989). More specifically, the more effective people are in resolving or coping with stressful problems in general, the more probable it is that they will not experience significant distress. Conversely, if a person has difficulty in coping with such difficulties, he or she will likely experience depression, anxiety, and other distress symptoms. Research that we, and others, have been conducting during the past two decades has provided substantial support for this general thesis (e.g., Kant, D'Zurilla, & Maydeu-Olivares, 1997; A. M. Nezu, Nezu, Saraydarian, Kalmar, & Ronan, 1986; A. M. Nezu & Ronan, 1985, 1988).

Given the plethora of problems that cancer patients experience, as delineated in the previous chapter, the applicability of the above-mentioned model to this population appeared obvious. In other words, we hypothesized that there would be a significant relationship between problem-solving ability and psychological distress among cancer patients. In addition, we believed that it was likely that effective problem-solving skills would serve to attenuate the deleterious effects of stress engendered by cancer and its treatment. Moreover, if these conjectures were valid, then teaching distressed cancer patients to become better at coping with stress would also be an effective intervention to help decrease their distress and to improve their overall quality of life.

This approach to understanding the stress–distress relationship among cancer patients is somewhat unique in that we emphasize the need to teach a *general coping approach* to individuals as compared with specific coping skills (see the Problem-Solving Coping section later in this chapter). Moreover, this approach is empirically derived and is based on a substantial body of clinically relevant research documenting the efficacy of problem-solving therapy. In addition, as underscored throughout this book, we emphasize the flexibility of this approach regarding patient population, method of implementation, and professional background of the problem-solving therapist.

Before we describe our problem-solving model of stress and coping, we begin this chapter with several definitions related to social problem solving and the overall problem-solving process. This is followed by a description of the problem-solving model of stress and coping and its relevance to the experience of cancer. Next, we review related research, in terms of both the validity of the model and the efficacy of problem-solving therapy itself.

Social Problem Solving

Our model of problem-solving training has historic roots stemming back over four decades, when various mental health professionals theorized that problem solving was positively related to social competence and was inversely related to psychopathology and maladaptive behavior. For example, Jahoda (1953) argued that problem-solving ability was a critical component of positive mental health and that deficits in problem-solving skills were associated with inadequate psychological adjustment and emotional distress. Since that time, substantial research has documented the existence of this relationship with regard to schizophrenia, depression, anxiety, substance abuse, stress, agoraphobia, obesity, and other clinical disorders (see D'Zurilla & Nezu, in press, for a comprehensive review of this literature).

In addition, important differences have been identified between individuals characterized as *effective* versus *ineffective* problem solvers. For example, effective problem solvers are more motivated to solve problems, have higher expectations of success, are less impulsive and avoidant, are more systematic and persistent, and have a clearer understanding of problems (Heppner, Hibel, Neal, Weinstein, & Rabinowitz, 1982) than do their ineffective counterparts. Effective problem solvers are also more assertive and less anxious (Neal & Heppner, 1982), have a more positive self-concept, have fewer dysfunctional thoughts and irrational beliefs (Heppner, Reeder, & Larson, 1983), and tend to use more rational decision-making strategies

(Phillips, Pazienza, & Ferrin, 1984) than do ineffective problem solvers.

Furthermore, when compared with effective problem solvers, ineffective problem solvers report a greater number of life problems (Heppner et al., 1982; A. M. Nezu, 1985), more health and physical symptoms (Sherry, Keitel, & Tracey, 1984), more anxiety (Neal & Heppner, 1982; A. M. Nezu, 1985, 1986d), more depression (Heppner, Baumgardner, & Jackson, 1985; Heppner, Kampa, & Brunning 1987; A. M. Nezu, 1985, 1986a; A. M. Nezu, Kalmar, Ronan, & Clavijo, 1986; A. M. Nezu, Nezu, et al., 1986; A. M. Nezu & Ronan, 1985), more psychological stress symptoms (Heppner et al., 1987), and more psychological maladjustment (Heppner & Anderson, 1985).

WHAT IS SOCIAL PROBLEM SOLVING?

In the literature regarding psychology and mental health, solving real-life problems has been referred to as *social problem solving, interpersonal problem solving, personal problem solving,* and *applied problem solving.* These differing terms highlight the personal and social context in which real-life problem solving takes place and differentiates this process from impersonal problem solving and general intelligence (A. M. Nezu et al., 1989). Although problem solving and general intellectual functioning are correlated, the actual strength of this relationship is minimal and, therefore, should not be viewed as synonymous (C. M. Nezu, Nezu, & Arean, 1991).

In their seminal article that synthesized the extant literature on problem solving at the time, D'Zurilla and Goldfried (1971) defined problem solving as "a behavioral process . . . which (a) makes available a variety of potentially effective response alternatives for dealing with a problematic situation, and (b) increases the probability of selecting the most effective response from among those alternatives" (p. 108). D'Zurilla and Nezu (1982) defined social problem solving as the "process whereby an individual identifies or discovers effective means of coping with problem situations encountered in day-to-day living" (p. 202). More in keeping with our problem-solving model of stress, as described later in this chapter, we define problem solving here as the process by which individuals understand the nature of problems in living and therefore direct their coping efforts at altering the problematic nature of the situations themselves, their reactions to them, or both (A. M. Nezu, 1987, 1989).

WHAT IS A PROBLEM?

Within this conceptualization, problems are defined as specific life circumstances that demand responses for adaptive functioning but that are not met with effective coping responses from the individuals confronted with them, because of the presence of various obstacles (D'Zurilla & Nezu, 1982). These obstacles may include ambiguity, uncertainty, conflicting demands, lack of resources, or novelty.

In essence, problems generally represent a discrepancy between the reality of a situation and one's desired goals (A. M. Nezu, 1987). These problems are likely to be stressful if they are at all difficult and relevant to one's well-being (D'Zurilla & Nezu, 1982). Problems can be single events (e.g., scheduling problems with a physician), a series of related events (e.g., negative side effects that are due to chemotherapy), or chronic situations (e.g., depressive reaction to cancer diagnosis and sexual difficulties resulting from cancer treatment). The demands in the problematic situation may originate in the environment (e.g., obstacles to overcome) or within the person (e.g., personal goals, needs, and commitments).

WHAT IS A SOLUTION?

In this model, a *solution* is defined as any coping response geared to modify the nature of the problematic situation, one's negative emotional reactions to it, or both (A. M. Nezu, 1987). *Effective solutions,* in particular, are those coping responses that not only achieve such goals but that also simultaneously maximize other positive consequences (i.e., benefits) and minimize other negative consequences (i.e., costs). These associated costs and benefits involve the short- and long-term effects of a solution plan, as well as both the personal consequences for the individual and the impact that the solution has on significant others.

It is important to note that the effectiveness of a given solution can vary from person to person and across differing settings for the same person because of differences in people's personal goals and values. For example, although many medical problems are often associated with similar solutions, depending on extenuating circumstances, adjustments often need to be made (e.g., varying medication doses that are due to differences in weight, sensitivity to side effects, and combinations with other medications). Psychosocial and emotional problems are even more variable across persons, even if they experience the same type of distress, such as depression or anxiety, because of differences in the cause of the distress (A. M. Nezu, Nezu, Friedman, & Haynes, 1997). Therefore, it is impossible to develop a cookbook of solutions to give to cancer patients that provide "advice–columnlike answers" to a catalog of difficulties. In other words, what might be an effective solution to one patient may not be helpful to another, hence the need for flexible problem-solving skills.

When discussing solutions, it is also important to differentiate between the concepts of problem solving and solution implementation (D'Zurilla & Nezu, in press). In essence, problem solving entails the process of discovery—the finding of an effective solution to a given problem. *Solution implementation,* on the other hand, refers to the actual carrying out of the solution or the coping *performance* of the chosen solution response. As such, coping performance refers to the outcome of the *problem-solving process,* suggesting that the term problem-solving coping represents the combination of problem solving and coping performance in response to a given stressful problem (A. M. Nezu et al., 1989). The distinction between problem solving and solution implementation is particularly important when an individual fails to resolve a problem effectively. To best assess "what went wrong," the problem-solving counselor needs to be able to differentiate between ineffective problem solving and actual deficits in the patient's performance skills. In addition, carrying out a solution plan is further dependent on emotional inhibitions and motivational limitations.

The Problem-Solving Process

PROBLEM ORIENTATION

Our definition of problem solving attempts to capture the importance of several key ideas. First, it highlights the notion that problem solving entails an overall psychological set or orientation that affects the manner in which people understand, think about, and react to problems in general. With regard to cancer, for example, common reactions are fear, anxiety, a general feeling of being overwhelmed, or a combination of all or some of these. This reaction is often not a result of direct experience, in which the newly diagnosed patient has a family member or close friend who has cancer. Instead, this reaction is often based on the general understanding or perception of cancer as "the big C" or as a leading cause of death.

We refer to this general perceptual set as *problem orientation.* This component differs from the other problem-solving variables in that it is a motivational process, whereas the other variables consist of specific skills and abilities that enable a person to solve a particular problem effectively. Problem orientation can be described as a set of orienting responses that represent the immediate cognitive–affective reactions of a person when first confronted with a problem. These orienting responses include a general sensitivity to problems, as well as various beliefs, assumptions, appraisals, and expectations concerning life's problems and one's own problem-solving abilities. If positive, one's orientation can engender positive affect and approach motivation, which in turn can facilitate effective problem solving. For example, among a sample of adult cancer patients, those characterized as having a positive problem orientation were found to be more optimistic about their future and reported lower levels of anxiety and depressive symptoms (Deaner, Nezu, & Nezu, 1997). A positive problem orientation has also been associated with optimism and positive affectivity in general (Chang & D'Zurilla, 1996) and more positive moods in times of challenge (Elliott, Sherwin, Harkins, & Marmarosh, 1995) and has been found to influence the manner in which people find meaning after the onset of a severe physical disability (Elliott & Johnson, 1995).

Conversely, a negative orientation can lead to negative affect, impulsive behavior, and avoidance motivation, which can inhibit or disrupt subsequent problem-solving attempts. For example, a negative problem orientation has been found to be associated with more negative moods under routine and stressful conditions and increases one's vulnerability to pessimism, negative emotional experiences, and clinical depression (e.g., Chang & D'Zurilla, 1996; Elliott et al., 1995; A. M. Nezu, 1987; Nezu et al., 1989). Furthermore, individuals with a negative orientation tend to worry (Dugas, Letarte, Rheaume, Freeston, & Ladoucer, 1995) and complain about their health (Godshall & Elliott, in press). In addition, caregivers of persons with recent-onset spinal cord injury report more anxiety, depression, and health complaints, regardless of the actual caregiving demands or severity of patient impairment, if their problem orientation is negative (Elliott, Shewchuk, Richards, Palmatier, & Margolis, 1997). A negative problem orientation has also been found to predict emotional distress among a sample of family caregivers of patients with Alzheimer's disease (Rothenberg, Nezu, Nezu, & Swain, 1994).

Training in the problem orientation component is geared to help individuals (a) increase their ability to recognize problems in living when they occur, (b) minimize the negative influence of immediate emotional distress and negative thoughts on further problem solving, (c) adopt the philosophical perspective that problems in living are commonplace and inevitable and that using a systematic approach to problem solving is an effective means of coping with them, (d) facilitate one's expectation of successful coping, and (e) inhibit the tendency to react impulsively or to avoid dealing with problems (A. M. Nezu et al., 1989). The orientation process includes five specific variables: problem perception, problem attribution, problem appraisal, personal control beliefs, and approach–avoidance style.

Problem Perception

This aspect of problem orientation involves the accurate recognition of stressful problems when they occur. Because of either a general tendency to avoid problems or an insensitivity to recognizing relevant information, when individuals do not identify a situation as a problem, they are ill prepared to deal with it effectively. Sensitivity to problems helps to spark the self-statement, "I need to do something about this situation," thereby facilitating future problem-solving activities (e.g., thinking of possible solutions or making decisions).

In addition to perceiving problems when they occur, it is important for the problem solver to label the *situation*, and not one's emotional response, as the problem. This helps the individual to later accurately identify what about the situation makes it a problem. Furthermore, emotions can often be used as cues or signals that a problem exists. In other words, rather than focusing on the problem of "feeling down in the dumps," the more effective view is to state that "feeling blue must mean that a problem exists." This increases the likelihood that the individual will attempt to identify accurately what is making him or her feel depressed and then seek to resolve it. At times, the changes may be external (e.g., change jobs), internal (e.g., improve job skills or change unrealistic goals), or both.

Problem Attribution

This orientation variable reflects the attributions of causality that people make regarding problems in living. One extreme is the tendency to make *internal* attributions such as the following: "It's always my fault, I'm just stupid!" or "It's my fault that I got cancer because I smoked too many cigarettes, I deserve this punishment." A general style that attributes the cause to stable internal factors can lead to maladaptive increases in responsibility, stress, and feelings of being overwhelmed. Moreover, such attributional biases can lead to ineffective attempts at problem-solving coping (Heppner et al., 1983). With regard to cancer, Watson, Greer, Prieyn, and Van Den Bourne (1990) found that patients who appeared to have an anxious preoccupation with their illness were more inclined to attribute the cause of the cancer to something within themselves.

An example of the other extreme are people who ascribe the cause of problems solely to external factors, such as other people, supervisors, institutions, or a supreme being. This type of attributional style also serves to inhibit later problem-solving activities: If the person generally attributes the reasons why a problem exists to external sources, the motivation to solve them diminishes greatly. As such, it is likely that problem gets worse and new problems arise.

Therefore, our problem-solving training model attempts to foster a willingness to engage in a reality-based search for the appropriate causes of a given problem. Given their complex nature, the causes of problems can at times be ascribed to the individual, at times to external factors, and often to a combination of both.

Problem Appraisal

This orientation aspect addresses differences in the way people evaluate the importance or significance of a given problem and its impact on one's overall well-being. One extreme is the judgment that a problem is trivial and has little effect, and the other extreme is the evaluation that the problem is a catastrophe and signals "doom." Research addressing the impact of stressful events points to the need to assess the *idiosyncratic* importance that an event has for a given individual (A. M. Nezu & Ronan, 1985). For example, the loss of a job to one person may be highly significant and stressful, whereas to another, it may not. Even the experience of cancer can have different meanings to different people, as well as different meanings for the same person across differing situations and over time (Thompson & Pitts, 1993).

In a study by Vinokur, Threatt, Vinokur-Kaplan, and Satariano (1990), appraisal of threat among a sample of breast cancer patients was significantly related to their degree of emotional distress. Moreover, the subjective appraisal of threat by the patient was found to be more influential in predicting distress than was the objective measure of the physician's prognosis.

Evaluating the importance of a problem can often be prone to error or even distortions, especially if one is already emotionally distressed. Specifically, as Beck, Rush, Shaw, and Emery (1979) noted, various errors in information processing can occur under stress, such as *magnification* and *minimization*. Magnification is the judgmental error that leads to an overemphasis of the importance of an essentially trivial event, whereas minimization involves the underestimation of the significance of an event when it is in fact important. Either misconception can lead to ineffective problem solving, especially when patients engender inaccurate definitions of the problem.

Personal Control Beliefs

People's beliefs regarding both the likelihood that a problem is solvable and that they are capable of effectively coping with the problem are important aspects of the problem orientation process (A. M. Nezu,

Kalmar, et al., 1986). The expectancy of being able to affect or control, at least in part, events that happen in one's life can help determine responses to problems. For example, Bloom and Broder (1950) found that successful problem solvers had greater confidence in their ability to solve the problems presented to them than did unsuccessful problem solvers. Effective problem solvers, compared with ineffective problem solvers, tend to view common life problems as being caused by *controllable* factors (Baumgardner, Heppner, & Arkin, 1986). Furthermore, research in general addressing the construct of locus of control consistently indicates that the overall expectation of being able to control one's environment greatly increases the probability that an individual will actively attempt to cope with stressful problems (Bandura, 1977; Rotter, 1966).

Conversely, extreme beliefs in one's ability to control the environment can also be detrimental to later problem-solving activities and consequent emotional reactions. Problem solving has been defined previously as a broad-based coping process, whereby possible effective solutions may be geared toward active attempts to change the problematic nature of the situation, one's emotional reaction to it, or both (A. M. Nezu, 1987). A person who defines successful solutions only as those that change the nature of the situation may encounter bitter disappointments, which can also lead to distress reactions. Believing at times that certain problems cannot be changed, such as a cancer diagnosis, allows the individual to also include emotion-focused goals as viable alternatives (e.g., acceptance and decrease in anxiety). As implied in our definition of problem solving, both goals are often relevant.

Related to this issue is the distinction noted by Thompson and Collins (1995) between primary and secondary control processes. Primary control consists of beliefs that one's actions can have a direct impact on a situation (e.g., improving one's diet can minimize the likelihood of cancer recurrence). Secondary control processes involve one's acceptance of the lack of control in a situation. Maladaptive examples of such processes include believing in luck or fate, whereas adaptive examples include anxiety reduction and reappraising the cancer diagnosis as a "wake-up call" requiring major lifestyle changes.

Approach–Avoidance Style

This last problem orientation variable addresses the manner in which individuals tend to either commit themselves to solving problems or deny or avoid their existence. Our bias is to state that, in general, it is better to approach or confront a problem than to avoid it. Denying that a problem exists only decreases the likelihood that the problem will be resolved and actually engenders the development of new problems. Avoiding problems can also disrupt later problem-solving activities. Heppner et al. (1983) found that ineffective problem solvers engaged in more irrational beliefs concerning problem avoidance as compared with effective problem solvers. In addition, avoidance of problems has been associated with greater alcohol consumption among college students (Godshall & Elliott, in press). Conversely, effective problem solvers more often consider effort to be an important determinant of their performance as compared with ineffective problem solvers (Baumgardner et al., 1986).

In a study with 603 cancer patients, Dunkel-Schetter, Feinstein, Taylor, and Falke (1992) found that cognitive (e.g., "Hoped a miracle would happen") and behavioral (e.g., "Avoided being with people") escape–avoidance coping patterns were associated with higher levels of emotional distress. In addition, extreme levels of denial can lead to significant delays in seeking medical treatment, which in turn have been found to have a devastating impact on the clinical course of those patients who come to the attention of a health professional only during later stages of cancer (Kunkel et al., 1997).

On the other hand, an extreme form of *approach behavior* can also be maladaptive. This occurs when an individual has the general tendency to solve problems impulsively, without taking the time or effort necessary to engage in planful and systematic problem solving. Because of previous experiences with similar problems, people may not "look before they leap" and attempt to implement a solution that may have worked in the past. Unless the situations are identical, it is likely that different aspects of the problem require different solutions. Therefore, our model posits that it is important for individuals, when confronted with stressful problems, to inhibit the tendency to respond impulsively and automatically. Rather, they should "stop and think."

The importance of this principle is highlighted in a study by Platt and Spivack (1974) that compared psychiatric patients with normal controls on a variety of problem-solving parameters. They found that control participants endorsed the idea that one needs to think before acting when providing solutions to hypothetical test problems. Conversely, the patient group showed more concern for taking immediate action. In addition, research by Bloom and Broder (1950) indicated that less successful problem solvers tend to be impulsive and impatient. Studies by Heppner and his colleagues (Heppner et al., 1982, 1983) additionally characterized effective problem solvers as being less impulsive, more insightful, and rating themselves as more likely to engage in and enjoy thinking.

Research on Training in Problem Orientation

Two studies highlight the importance of emphasizing the problem orientation component in problem-solving training. First, in an investigation by Cormier, Otani, and Cormier (1986), participants who received instructions in this component performed significantly better than control participants on two subsequent problem-solving tasks. One task involved selecting the best alternative from a list of possible solutions, whereas the second measure required participants to describe actual behaviors used to solve a series of six interpersonal problems.

One purpose of an outcome study by A. M. Nezu and Perri (1989) involved testing the relative contribution of the problem orientation component in treating clinically depressed adults. A dismantling strategy was used to address this goal by randomly assigning a group of diagnosed depressed participants to one of three conditions: problem-solving therapy (PST; training in the entire model), abbreviated problem-solving therapy (APST; entire model minus training in the orientation process), and waiting-list control (WLC). Results indicated that although APST participants reported significantly lower posttreatment depression scores than WLC members, PST participants evidenced significantly lower levels of depressive symptomatology at posttreatment than both the APST and WLC participants. It was concluded that although APST members were taught various problem-solving coping skills (i.e., defining problems, generating alternative solutions, and decision making), not specifically addressing their problem-solving set may have led to less effective treatment.

RATIONAL PROBLEM-SOLVING SKILLS

Our definition of problem solving also emphasizes the act of directing various coping efforts toward problem resolution or the act of changing the nature of the situation so that it is no longer problematic. Identification of such effective and appropriate solutions or coping efforts is achieved through specific problem-solving tasks, known as *rational problem-solving skills.* These involve a group of specific skills or goal-directed tasks that enable a person to solve a particular problem successfully and can be defined as the rational, planful, systematic, and skillful application of various effective problem-solving principles and techniques. Each task makes a distinct contribution toward the discovery of an adaptive solution or coping response in a problem-solving situation.

These four skill domains include *problem definition* and *formulation* (i.e., ability to understand the nature of a problem, identify obstacles to goals, delineate realistic objectives, and perceive cause–effect relationships), *generation of alternatives* (i.e., ability to brainstorm multiple solution ideas), *decision making* (i.e., ability to identify potential consequences, predict the likelihood of such consequences, and conduct a cost–benefit analysis of desirability of these outcomes), and *solution implementation* and *verification* (i.e., ability to carry out a solution optimally, monitor its effects, troubleshoot if solution is not effective, and self-reinforce if outcome is satisfactory).

Problem Definition and Formulation

The purpose of this problem-solving process is to assess accurately the nature of a problem and to identify realistic goals. Its importance for guiding latter problem-solving activities is paramount. To paraphrase a quote from John Dewey (1910), "A problem well defined is half solved." In a variety of empirical evaluations, training individuals to develop well-defined problems has been found to have a positive impact on later problem-solving tasks, such as generating quality solutions and making effective decisions (Cormier et al., 1986; Hansen, St. Lawrence, & Christoff, 1985; A. Nezu & D'Zurilla, 1981a, 1981b). In real-life situations, stressful problems are usually complex and ambiguous. Therefore, training in this initial problem-solving task encourages people to (a) seek all available facts and information about a problem, (b) describe such facts in clear language, (c) differentiate relevant from irrelevant information and objective facts from assumptions, (d) identify the factors and circumstances that make the situation a problem, and (e) set realistic problem-solving goals.

Obtain Information

Rarely do problems in living come in "neat packages." Often, individuals need to obtain additional information about a problem, especially when it is complex. Attempting to understand the exact nature of a stressful problem without gathering information is similar to a health professional diagnosing a patient without the benefit of conducting tests or gathering data from clinical interviews. As such, the problem solver is encouraged to gather information in an attempt to gain a "complete picture."

Use Clear Language

The use of concrete, clear, and unambiguous terms can help minimize confusion and misperceptions about the nature of a problem. Stating the problem specifically and concretely helps an individual to make relevant what may have appeared initially to be irrelevant, thus increasing the likelihood of effective problem solving. Bloom and Broder (1950), for example, found that successful problem solvers tended to translate difficult and unfamiliar terms into simpler, more concrete language. On the other hand, unsuccessful problem solvers tended to accept vague concepts without attempting to reformulate them into more understandable terms.

Minimize Misperceptions and Cognitive Distortions

In attempts to define a problem, individuals at times may use information that is based on inaccurate judgments, assumptions, and interpretations. The more stressful and complex a problem is, the higher the likelihood that an individual may make errors in information processing. In such cases, it is likely that individuals will attempt to solve "pseudoproblems" instead of real problems because the problem conceptualization is inaccurate. These pseudoproblems are unsolvable because solutions identified to deal with them are likely to be inappropriate or irrelevant for the actual problem. In addition, as noted earlier, various cognitive distortions, such as magnification, can influence the process of accurately defining a problem. Furthermore, selectively attending to negative aspects of a problem can also lead to inaccurate problem conceptualization.

Another type of cognitive error can occur while the person is engaged in means–end thinking. Means–end thinking refers to the process of identifying cause–effect relationships and anticipating the consequences of a solution. In particular, such an error occurs when the problem solver overestimates or underestimates the probability that a particular effect will follow a certain event or that certain consequences will result as a function of certain behaviors. As Rehm (1981) noted, depressed individuals characteristically show selective attention to immediate consequences instead of long-range effects. Errors in over- or underestimating the impact of certain consequences may also result in the creation of pseudoproblems.

Identify Why a Problem Is a Problem

This aspect of the problem-definition-and-formulation component is perhaps the most difficult. It is during this process that individuals begin to use the information previously gathered as a means of formulating why a given situation is a problem. We defined a problem earlier as "a discrepancy between the demands of a situation and the availability of effective responses." In essence, then, the problem solver at this juncture is attempting to identify specifically what it is about the situation that causes this discrepancy. Posing the following types of questions helps this process: "What are the conditions that are getting me upset?" "What would I like to have happen?" "What are the changes necessary to reach my goals?" "What are the obstacles that I have to overcome in order to reach these goals?" "Who is creating these obstacles?" "Are there any conflicts involved?" and "Who do these conflicts involve?"

Often the answers to such questions fall into one of the following four categories of reasons why a problem is a problem: (a) *presence of a threat or aversive stimuli* (e.g., arguments with one's spouse, getting fired from a job, failing an exam, receiving a severe traffic violation, getting rejected when asking for a date, and prolonged medical complications), (b) *loss of positive experiences* (e.g., death of a family member, unwanted divorce or separation, loss of a close friend who moves away, unexpected limitation in various abilities, decreased finances, job demotion, and aging), (c) *presence of obstacles* (e.g., lack of resources, limited finances, limited skills, and emotional distress), and (d) *presence of conflicts* (e.g., differences in goals within a person and conflicts in opinions or interests between people).

In addition, problems can vary in their degree of novelty, magnitude of seriousness, complexity, and depth. Unfamiliar or novel situations are likely to be particularly stressful because they involve aspects of uncertainty. As the degree of unfamiliarity of a situation increases, so does the number of decisions that need to be made. This often requires more active and concerted attempts at problem solving and an increased vigilance toward adopting the problem-solving set of "problems in living are normal and inevitable."

Problems can also vary regarding the magnitude of actual and potential negative consequences. Assessment of this component of a problem requires an appreciation of both immediate and long-term effects of a problem, which can help the problem solver to eventually develop a time plan for achieving various subgoals and objectives.

Problems also differ in complexity. Complex problems often involve situations that either overlap with other significant problems or encompass a group of several smaller problems. With regard to the former, it is important for the problem solver to understand how one problem may be intertwined with another. In such cases, the consequences of one situation can have a great bearing on the effects of the second. With regard to the second type, the problem solver needs to break the complex problem into smaller, more manageable ones.

Problems can also vary in terms of depth. Because there are several ways that any particular problem can be defined and formulated, different individuals may focus on varying levels of the problem. The real problem is the one that is primary, basic, or fundamental. It might be the first problem in a chain of events. For example, children may react to a parent's cancer diagnosis with fear, anxiety, and feelings of hopelessness. However, such a reaction in children often manifests itself in lowered school performance and increased behavioral problems, which in turn may lead to increased friction between parent and child, which can then engender poor family communication patterns (i.e., Problem A causes Problem B, which causes Problem C, and so forth). Instead of focusing only on the problem of the child's behavior problems, it is more effective to also address the original problem of the child's fears. The success of any solution implemented to resolve Problem C or Problem D may thus only be short-lived. Furthermore, resolving Problem A may also resolve the remaining problems.

The real problem may also involve a larger, broader situation. By focusing on only one part of a problem, people often develop solutions that ultimately fail. Other conflicts or obstacles that remain unattended to can lead to ineffective solutions. Especially when a problem is complex, the individual needs to formulate the "big picture." Such a conceptualization of a problem situation requires awareness of both the "forest" and the "trees."

Setting Goals

In general, goals involve descriptions of the desired outcome of a problem. However, as defined earlier, an effective solution not only changes the nature of the situation so that it is no longer a problem but, in addition, also maximizes associated positive consequences and minimizes any negative consequences. Therefore, goals should also entail statements concerning the overall desired outcome. Furthermore, in specifying goals, the problem solver needs to avoid stating goals that are unrealistic or irrational. Unrealistic goals actually change the problem from a potentially solvable one to an insoluble situation, as they are impossible to attain. Furthermore, the impact on one's orientation (e.g., personal control beliefs) can be substantial. In other words, attempts to reach an unattainable goal are doomed to fail. Such unsuccessful attempts can then reinforce one's negative orientation regarding a limited ability to cope with the problem and can even lead to generalized beliefs about uncontrollability in general. With regard to cancer, for example, Wan, Counte, and Cella (1997) suggested that patients would benefit from being encouraged to set and maintain realistic goals concerning their cancer prognosis and treatment process.

Goals should be stated in the form of "How can I _____?" or "What can be done to _____?" For example, "How can I get more people to visit me at home while I am so tired by the chemotherapy—

I feel so lonely?" or "What can be done so that I don't feel so hopeless about the future?" With complex problems, various subgoals should be specified to address the "various trees within the larger forest."

In setting goals, the problem solver now has the opportunity to reappraise or evaluate the overall nature of the problem regarding its importance and significance for well-being. With vague and undefined problems, the individual may have previously perceived the problem to be quite threatening and hopeless. After clarifying the nature of the situation, it may be possible that a more complete picture emerges, and the problem is then perceived as more manageable.

Generation of Alternatives

After defining a problem and setting realistic goals, the problem solver is ready to generate alternative solutions. Training in this problem-solving component is geared to help individuals think of a wide range of possible alternative ideas to solve the problem in order to maximize the likelihood that the best or most effective solution ideas will be eventually identified. Underlying this approach is the brainstorming procedure, which was originally developed to facilitate "idea finding" among groups and has widely been used in industrial and management settings (Parnes, 1967). Brainstorming incorporates three general principles: (a) the quantity principle, (b) the deferment-of-judgment principle, and (c) the strategies and tactics principle. With specific regard to real-life problems, research has indicated that training individuals to use these principles increases their ability to think of effective solutions to real-life problems (D'Zurilla & Nezu, 1980; A. Nezu & D'Zurilla, 1981b; A. M. Nezu & Ronan, 1987).

Quantity Principle

The first brainstorming principle, the quantity principle, suggests that the more alternative solutions that individuals generate, the more likely they are to arrive at the potentially best ideas for a solution. In studies by Parnes (1967) and Maier and Hoffman (1964), participants who followed brainstorming instructions tended to contribute significantly more effective ideas to the last half of a list, as compared with the first half, as they were able to be more creative as they continued to engage in the task.

Deferment-of-Judgment Principle

This second brainstorming principle, deferment of judgment, posits that more high-quality ideas can be produced if an individual defers critical evaluation of any idea until after a comprehensive list of possibilities has been compiled. In other words, during this phase of problem-solving training, individuals are taught to withhold judgment about any of the ideas. Consideration of the value, effectiveness, or moral acceptability of an alternative is avoided at this juncture, with the exception of the one requirement that the idea be relevant to the problem. Premature evaluation of the alternatives leads to a restricted range of ideas.

Strategies and Tactics Procedure

This last brainstorming principle, strategies and tactics strategy, suggests that individuals should first think of *general means* or *strategies* to solve a problem and subsequently produce various *tactics* or *specific ways* in which a strategy might be implemented. In this manner, a greater variety or range of ideas might be produced, which can also increase the overall generation of ideas.

The use of these general approaches to idea production also serves to inhibit impulsivity. Under stressful situations, some individuals may attempt to cope by engaging in previously successful solutions without analyzing whether it is appropriate to do so. As noted earlier, unless the current problem is exactly the same as the previous one, impulsive attempts are likely to fail.

In addition to these three principles, training in this component emphasizes the use of concrete and unambiguous language when describing or delineating various alternative solutions. The problem solver can also increase the effectiveness of brainstorming by attempting to (a) generate combinations of ideas, (b) modify and improve on certain alternatives, (c) elaborate on previously generated ideas, or (d) use any or all of these (D'Zurilla & Nezu, in press).

Decision Making

Having generated a wide range of alternative solution ideas, the problem solver must now evaluate each possibility and select the most effective one(s) for implementation. The primary focus at this point is the assessment of a given alternative with regard to its consequences. Our training approach to this process draws heavily on *utility theory* (Edwards, Lindman, & Phillips, 1965), which represents a means–end conceptualization of decision theory, in which the expected utility of a given alternative is defined as a joint function of both the *value* of each outcome and the *likelihood* that a given alternative will achieve a given result. In essence, individuals are trained to conduct a cost–benefit analysis regarding the consequences of a given solution. Training individuals in this model of decision making has been shown to be highly efficacious with specific regard to real-life problems in a variety of studies (Cormier et al., 1986; A. Nezu & D'Zurilla, 1979, 1981a; A. M. Nezu & Ronan, 1987).

Estimates of Likelihood of Effects

The first assessment that the problem solver makes involves an estimate of the likelihood that a given alternative will have a particular effect. In essence, this probability evaluation addresses the question of whether the alternative will meet the problem-solving goals previously delineated (i.e., "Will it work?"). In addition, our model suggests that an assessment of the likelihood that the problem solver can actually carry out the alternative in its optimal form is of equal importance. A given solution might theoretically be an excellent idea, but may be less than optimal in reality because of limitations of the problem solver's ability to carry it out. The individual in the situation must therefore undergo a personal assessment of his or her assets and liabilities to determine the feasibility of a given alternative.

Estimates of Value

In making judgments about the value of an alternative, four categories of consequences should be considered: short-term or immediate consequences, long-term consequences, personal consequences (effects on oneself), and social consequences (effects on others). Personal consequences involve the time and effort required to implement a particular alternative, personal and emotional costs or gains, consistency with one's ethical and moral standards, and physical well-being. Within the social category, specific outcomes may include effects on one's family, friends, or community.

Because people differ in their personal values, goals, and commitments, it is impossible to develop a standard set of consequences for each type of problematic situation. As such, it is important for the individual problem solver to brainstorm the myriad of potential outcomes associated with a given alternative.

On the basis of this cost–benefit analysis, the problem solver is able to identify those ideas for which the expected overall outcome most closely matches the problem-solving goals. If only a few alternatives appear to be potentially satisfactory, then the problem solver must consider several questions: "Do I have enough information about the problem?" "Did I define the problem correctly?" "Are my goals too high?" and "Did I generate enough options?" At this juncture, then, the individual is directed to go back and engage in the previous problem-solving tasks.

Conversely, the individual who has identified a variety of satisfactory alternatives is encouraged to develop an overall solution plan. This is accomplished by combining several potentially effective coping options for each subgoal in order to attack the problem from various perspectives. Furthermore, the problem solver is encouraged to develop a contingency or backup plan in case the original ideas do not work.

Solution Implementation and Verification

At this stage, the problem solver is ready to implement the solution plan. Rather than simply carrying the solution out and "moving on," individuals need to compare the actual outcome of the solution with the anticipated ones. Even though a problem may be solved symbolically, the effectiveness of a solution has not yet been established. By carrying out the coping response, it is possible to evaluate the outcome and to verify its effectiveness.

In helping the problem solver to determine whether the match between the anticipated consequences and the actual consequences is good, we draw heavily on self-control theory (Kanfer, 1970), which involves four tasks: (a) behavioral performance, (b) self-monitoring, (c) self-evaluation, and (d) self-reinforcement. Within our problem-solving framework, this procedure therefore entails carrying out a solution, observing the actual consequences of that solution, evaluating the effectiveness of the solution, and reinforcing oneself if the problem becomes resolved.

Carrying Out the Solution Plan

The performance aspect of this process is the actual implementation of one's solution plan. As noted earlier, problem-solving performance can be influenced by factors other than one's problem-solving ability, such as specific skill deficits, emotional inhibitions, and motivational difficulties. Although these types of obstacles should have been identified during the decision-making process (i.e., the likelihood that the individual within the problem can actually implement the chosen solution in its optimal form), at times it is impossible to anticipate such consequences. The problem solver who discovers immediately that such performance problems exist should engage in either of two strategies: (a) return to the previous problem-solving tasks, such as generating alternatives and decision making, to identify a different solution plan or (b) reformulate the overall problem to include a subgoal for overcoming the obstacles related to effective coping performance.

Monitoring the Solution Outcome

This process often entails measuring the consequences of the solution outcome at varying levels. To obtain accurate information concerning the outcome, it may be necessary to identify or even develop an objective procedure to record such details. Similar to health professionals who continue to monitor the effects of a given medical procedure, we suggest the need to monitor the consequences of solution plans for personal problems.

Evaluating the Solution Outcome and Self-Reinforcement

In the evaluation step, the problem solver compares the actual outcome with the desired outcome that was specified during the problem-definition-and-formulation process (i.e., the problem-solving goal). If the match is satisfactory, then the individual moves to the last step, *self-reinforcement.* In other words, the individual should also reward problem resolution as "a job well-done." Such self-reinforcement can include simple positive self-statements, tangible gifts, or rewards (i.e., dining at an expensive restaurant or buying a new article of clothing). The actual resolution of the problem in itself can be an important source of reinforcement, especially if it engenders additional social reinforcement, reduction of aversive stimulation, removal of an obstacle to a goal, or resolution of a conflict. However, the self-reinforcement step is also crucial for the overall problem-solving process for two reasons: (a) It reinforces effective problem-solving coping and (b) it strengthens perceived self-control and self-efficacy expectations, which also affect future problem-solving efforts.

Conversely, if the match between the observed outcome and the problem-solving goal(s) is not satisfactory, the problem solver needs to discover the source of this discrepancy. This gap may have resulted because of difficulties in the problem-solving process, the performance of the solution response, or both. If it involves the first, the problem solver should "recycle" and return to one or more of the previous operations and attempt to discover another, more effective solution plan. If the discrepancy resulted from the less than optimal solution implementation, the problem solver faces the choice of either attempting to improve the performance or going through the problem-solving process once more to determine differing coping responses that may permit better implementation. Improving one's performance might require behavioral rehearsal of the skills used in the solution plan, reducing the inhibitory effects of emotional arousal that affect optimal coping performance, or providing more self-incentives or self-reinforcement. Which strategy to take depends on the actual factors interfering with the performance.

Problem-Solving Model of Stress and Coping

The rationale underlying the applicability of PST to help improve the quality of life of cancer patients is embedded within our problem-solving model of stress (A. M. Nezu, Nezu, Houts, Friedman, & Faddis, in press). As depicted in Figure 2.1, stress, within this model, is defined by the reciprocal relationships among major negative life events, daily problems, negative emotional states, and problem-solving coping (A. Nezu & D'Zurilla, 1989; A. M. Nezu et al., 1989).

FIGURE 2.1

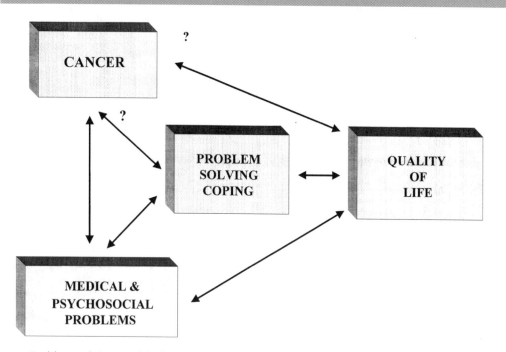

Problem-solving model of stress and coping: Reciprocal relationships among major negative life events, daily problems, negative emotional states, and problem-solving coping.

CANCER AS A MAJOR NEGATIVE LIFE EVENT

Over the last several decades, a plethora of research has documented the influence of major negative life events in causing psychological distress (A. M. Nezu & Ronan, 1985). Such events include divorce, death of a family member, losing a job, getting into a major traffic accident, and chronic illness. The experience of cancer can easily be characterized as a major negative life stressor that often engenders psychological distress and decreased quality of life (Jacobsen & Holland, 1991). The psychosocial consequences of cancer and its treatment were reviewed in detail in chapter 1.

CANCER-RELATED PROBLEMS AS A SECOND SOURCE OF STRESS

In addition, major stressful events, in general, create and increase the frequency of minor life events, hassles, or daily problems that also require a coping response (A. M. Nezu, 1986b; A. M. Nezu & Ronan, 1985). For example, in addition to the obvious medical issues, having cancer can result in a myriad of significant minor problems, such as financial difficulties, feelings of isolation, loneliness, family difficulties, depression, anxiety, and work difficulties. As Schag, Heinrich, Aadland, and Ganz (1990) noted, "patients are living for extended periods of time, thus being forced to cope with the chronic debilitating effects of cancer and its treatment, affecting all areas of functioning: physical, psychological, social and vocational . . . cancer patients have a variety of day-to-day problems and rehabilitation needs" (p. 84). Research has demonstrated that minor life events or problems have been found to be strongly related to psychological symptomatology, possibly even more so than major stressful life events (Monroe, 1983; A. M. Nezu & Ronan, 1985). As such, both major negative life events and daily problems can lead to psychological distress and poor quality of life, as noted in Figure 2.1.

Problems can also develop independent of major life changes, as a normal part of daily living. Furthermore, the accumulation of daily problems can result in a major life change, which, in turn, produces additional new daily problems (A. M. Nezu, 1986b; A. M. Nezu & Ronan, 1985). Major stressful life events and daily problems therefore function to influence each other in a reciprocal fashion, potentially creating ever-increasing stressful effects. With regard to cancer, for example, severe medical complications or negative side effects resulting from cancer treatment regimens can have an adverse effect on one's overall health outcome; hence, the bidirectionality of the arrows between cancer and related problems, as depicted in Figure 2.1.

PSYCHOLOGICAL DISTRESS AND DECREASED QUALITY OF LIFE

Psychological distress, such as depression and anxiety, can occur as a consequence of (a) particular negative conditions inherent in the problem, such as harm or pain, ambiguity, conflict, novelty, and complexity; (b) one's appraisal of the problem as a threat, a poor self-assessment of ability to cope with the threat; (c) ineffective attempts at problem solving; or (d) as a result of one or any of these. As noted in chapter 1, substantial psychosocial consequences can occur as a result of cancer and its treatment.

Whether psychological distress, such as depression, has a direct effect on cancer health outcome remains a controversial, but empirical, question (Watson & Ramirez, 1991); hence the presence of a question mark in Figure 2.1 near the arrow going from quality of life to cancer. It is important to note, however, that we are not suggesting that psychological factors are influential regarding the pathophysiology or biology of cancer *onset*, but rather that such variables can affect the *course* of the disease (Fox, 1983). For example, research has provided support for the relationship between various psychosocial variables and cancer *prognosis*, such as helplessness (Pettingale, Morris, Greer, & Haybittle, 1985) and depressed mood (Temoshok, 1985).

PROBLEM-SOLVING COPING

Continued successful coping attempts serve to reduce or minimize one's immediate emotional distress (e.g., depressive *symptomatology*) in reaction to a stressful event, as well as attenuate the probability of long-term negative outcomes (e.g., depressive *disorder* and poor quality of life). However, if one's coping skills are ineffective, or if extreme emotional distress negatively affects one's coping efforts, resulting in reduced motivation, inhibition of problem-solving performance, or both, then the likelihood of long-term negative affective conditions or poor overall quality of life would be increased. These negative outcomes can then increase the number of daily problems, the severity of daily problems, or both. For example, depression reduces motivation for active attempts at complying with medical treatment; this, in turn, may lead to another major life change or loss, such as poor health outcome.

According to Lazarus and Folkman (1984), the term *coping* refers to the cognitive and behavioral activities by which a person attempts to manage a trying situation. They have identified two general forms of coping: problem-focused coping and emotion-focused coping. *Problem-focused coping* is aimed at changing the objective problematic situation (i.e., the imbalance between demands and adaptive response availability) for the better, whereas *emotion-focused coping* is aimed at managing the emotional distress that is associated with the problem. Lazarus and Folkman view problem solving as a form of problem-focused coping in which the adaptive utility is limited to problematic situations that are appraised as changeable. On the other hand, when a stressful situation is appraised as *unchangeable,* the individual must rely on emotion-focused forms of coping in order to manage stress effectively.

In our model, problem-solving coping has more adaptive versatility than that characterized by Lazarus and Folkman (1984) because problem-solving goals may include problem-focused goals, emotion-focused goals, or both, depending on the nature of the problem and how it is appraised (A. M. Nezu & D'Zurilla, 1989). For example, problem-focused goals would be emphasized in problematic situations that are appraised as potentially changeable (e.g., negative side effects that are due to radiation treatment), although emotion-focused goals may also be included when emotional stress is high (i.e., distress associated with these negative side effects). In situations such as poor cancer prognosis that are appraised as initially unchangeable, emotion-focused goals such as acceptance would be more desirable. In cases in which the problematic situation is appraised initially as changeable, but because of unsuccessful coping attempts is later reappraised as unchangeable, the problem can then be reformulated to include emotion-focused goals, such as minimizing emotional distress, enhancing personal growth, or maintaining a sense of self-worth. Thus, we view problem-solving coping as a *general coping approach* that can help people manage or adapt to any stressful situation, thereby enhancing flexibility and perceived control, as well as minimizing emotional distress, even in situations that cannot be changed for the better (D'Zurilla & Nezu, in press; A. M. Nezu et al., 1989). Given the complex psychosocial context surrounding the experience of cancer, such flexibility is especially important.

Similar to the direct effect of quality of life on cancer health outcome, the question of whether psychosocial interventions improve survival rates is also controversial and unanswered. Although some studies indicate that improved psychosocial functioning is associated with longer survival rates, reduced mortality rates, or both (e.g., Fawzy et al., 1990; Richardson, Shelton, Krailo, & Levine, 1990; Spiegel, Bloom, Kraemer, & Gottheil, 1989), others provide contradictory findings (Cassileth, Walsh, & Lusk, 1988; Jamison, Burish, & Wallston, 1987). A complete discussion of this complex issue is beyond the scope of this book. However, as described in chapter 1, the experience of cancer can have a devastating impact on one's quality of life. Empirically based psychosocial interventions, such as problem-solving therapy, can have an enormous positive influence on the overall life of the cancer patient. Moreover, because of the lack of well-controlled, large-scale outcome studies geared to specifically address the issue of improved survival rates, this question remains empirical (see Dreher, 1997).

In summary, each of the four major stress-related variables (major negative life events, daily problems, psychological distress, and problem-solving coping) influences the others either to escalate the stress process and eventually produce clinically significant psychological disorders and poor quality of life or to reduce it and attenuate these negative long-term effects. The type of outcome that results depends on the nature of these four variables as they interact and change over time (A. M. Nezu, 1987; A. M. Nezu et al., 1989). Therefore, we place key emphasis on problem-solving therapy as a means of affecting this stress process in order to facilitate problem-solving effectiveness as a means of improving one's coping ability and to reduce emotional distress.

Research Support of the Model

For our problem-solving model to be tenable, three general research questions must be answered positively:

1. Is there a significant inverse relationship between problem solving and psychological distress?
2. Do effective problem-solving skills attenuate distress engendered by stressful events? and
3. Do therapeutic interventions that are based on problem-solving training lead to meaningful reductions in distress?

PROBLEM SOLVING AND DISTRESS

With regard to the first question, research has documented the existence of a strong association between problem-solving deficits and psychological distress. With regard to depression, for example, several investigators found depressed individuals to be less effective problem solvers than their nondepressed counterparts (Gotlib & Asarnow, 1979; A. M. Nezu, 1986a; A. M. Nezu & Ronan, 1987; Sacco & Graves, 1984; Zemore & Dell, 1983). Furthermore, poor problem solvers, as compared with effective problem solvers, have been found to report higher levels of depression across a variety of depression assessment procedures (Heppner & Anderson, 1985; Heppner et al., 1985; Heppner et al., 1987). Poor problem solving has also been found to be positively related to anxiety (A. M. Nezu, 1986d; A. M. Nezu & Carnevale, 1987).

Recently, we reported the results of two studies more directly assessing the association between problem-solving coping and cancer-related distress (C. M. Nezu et al., in press). The first study included 35 men and 70 women (mean age = 48.5 years) who were diagnosed with cancer within 1 year of their participation in this study. Diagnoses included the following major cancer types: leukemia (28%), breast (41%), colon (4%), ovarian (4%), cervical (2%), non-Hodgkin's lymphoma (5%), and other (colon, prostrate, bladder, and rectal; 16%). Approximately 83% were White, 13% African American, 1% Asian, and 3% Hispanic. Participants completed the following self-report inventories: the Social Problem-Solving Inventory—Revised (SPSI–R; D'Zurilla, Nezu, & Maydeu-Olivares, in press), the Brief Symptom Inventory (BSI; Derogatis & Spencer, 1982), and the Cancer Rehabilitation Evaluation System—Research Form (CARES; Schag & Heinrich, 1989).

The SPSI–R is a 52-item self-report inventory that measures social problem solving across five dimensions: (a) *negative problem orientation* (NPO; general set to view problems as threats, expect problems to be unsolvable, doubt one's own ability to solve problems successfully, and become frustrated and upset when experiencing problems); (b) *positive problem orientation* (PPO; general set to appraise problems as challenges, be optimistic in believing that problems are solvable, perceive one's own ability to solve problems as high, believe that successful problem solving involves time and effort, and be willing to commit oneself to confronting rather than avoiding problems); (c) *rational problem solving* (RPS; rational, systematic, and skillful application of various effective problem-solving strategies, such as concretely defining problem-solving goals, systematically searching for information, discriminating between facts and assumptions, generating large numbers of alternative solutions, conducting a systematic cost–benefit analysis of the various alternatives when making decisions, monitoring the outcome of one's solution, and comparing expected outcomes with actual outcomes); (d) *impulsivity–carelessness style* (ICS; a generalized problem-solving style characterized by impulsive, hurried, and careless attempts at problem resolution); and (e) *avoidance style* (AS; a second maladaptive problem-solving style characterized by procrastination, passivity, and dependency).

The BSI is a 53-item self-report measure of psychological distress symptoms experienced by both medical and psychiatric patients and has been shown to be especially useful for cancer patients (Zabora, Smith-Wilson, Fetting, & Enterline, 1990). Two of the BSI subscales were used in this study—Depression and Anxiety—as they represent the more typical psychosocial reaction to stressful events. The Depression subscale contains 6 items that reflect various aspects of clinical depression (e.g., feelings of hopelessness and dysphoric mood). The Anxiety subscale also contains 6 items and includes symptoms and signs associated with high levels of manifest anxiety (e.g., feeling fearful, signs of nervousness, and tension).

The CARES is a cancer-specific measure designed to assess day-to-day problems and rehabilitation needs of cancer patients. Because it represents a comprehensive list of problems encountered by cancer patients as they cope with the disease and its treatment on a daily basis, the CARES was included in this study as a measure of their overall quality of life. The total score was used as the measure of interest in this study.

A canonical correlational analysis was used to assess the relationship between psychological distress and social problem solving among the 105 adult cancer patients. In this analysis, the five scale scores of the SPSI–R represented various components of the construct of problem solving, whereas psychological distress was operationally defined by the Depression and Anxiety subscales of the BSI, in addition to the total CARES score. Results indicated that participants who were characterized by less effective problem-solving ability in general (i.e., high negative orientation, low positive orientation, low rational problem solving, high impulsive/carelessness style, and high avoidance style) were also found to report higher levels of depressive and anxiety symptomatology, as well as greater numbers of cancer-related problems.

In the second investigation, we were interested in determining whether problem solving served as a predictor of psychological distress years after successful breast cancer surgery (C. M. Nezu et al., in press). As such, our participants included 64 women who had successfully undergone surgery for breast cancer. Approximately 39% underwent a mastectomy, with the remainder receiving lumpectomies. The mean age of this group of participants was approximately 54 years, and the number of years since surgery ranged between 1.00 and 13.30 years ($M = 5.01$ years). In addition to surgery to remove the tumor, all of the women also received additional forms of medical treatment (45% received chemotherapy, 30% received radiation therapy, and 25% received both).

In essence, we conducted two separate multiple regression analyses in which the dependent variables included the Anxiety and Depression scales of the BSI (see above). Predictor variables included (a) the amount of time since surgery, (b) the five scales of the SPSI–R (i.e., NPO, PPO, RPS, ICS, and AS), and (c) a demographic variable representing additional medical treatment (i.e., chemotherapy, radiation therapy, or both). In addition, the effects of current stress unrelated to breast cancer (e.g., financial difficulties or recent loss of a family member) in predicting distress were controlled for by including a measure of current negative life stress as a covariate (the Life Experiences Survey; Sarason, Johnson, & Siegel, 1978).

Results indicated that NPO and RPS were found to be significant predictors of distress beyond that accounted for by current stressors among the sample of breast cancer survivors. Moreover, the amount of time that passed since surgery did not appear to be correlated with distress levels. It therefore appears that time per se did not "heal all wounds" and that the effectiveness of an individual's problem-solving ability was found to be an important dimension in determining quality of life.

A study that addressed the relationship between problem solving and distress with specific regard to sexual dysfunctions involved adults who underwent a bone marrow transplant (BMT) and high-dose chemotherapy, as several studies have suggested that such treatment may be associated with a variety of psychological difficulties including sexual problems (A. M. Nezu & Nezu, 1998). As part of a larger study (Marks, Crilley, Nezu, & Nezu, 1996), 30 participants completed several measures, including the SPSI–R and the Derogatis Interview for Sexual Functioning—Self-Report Version (DISF; Derogatis, 1986) at baseline and at 3 months post-BMT. This latter measure provides a self-report assessment of overall sexual functioning with different versions for men and women. The median age of this sample was 38 years, and over 90% were White and over 60% were married. This sample also represents inpatients undergoing consecutive BMT therapy for cancer who gave informed consent. Fifteen participants received an autograft BMT, whereas 12 received an allograft, and 3 were in the unrelated donor category.

To determine whether problem solving predicts sexual dysfunction post-BMT, A. M. Nezu and Nezu (1998) conducted a multiple regression analysis, whereby post-BMT DISF scores served as the dependent variable and pre-BMT SPSI–R total scores served as the primary predictor. In addition, pre-BMT DISF scores served as a covariate. Results indicated that after partialing out the effects due to previous sexual functioning, problem solving significantly predicted post-BMT sexual dysfunction. In other words, the quality and effectiveness of one's problem-solving skills appear to be operative in determining sexual satisfaction, dysfunction, or both, that might ensue as a result of a BMT.

Although they do not directly assess problem-solving abilities as defined earlier, studies that focus on coping and cancer provide collaborative support of our overall model. For example, in a review of such studies, Rowland (1990a) identified the following common themes that cut across varying cancer populations, disease sites, and assessment methods: (a) Strategies that promote active problem-solving and coping behaviors are consistently found to be the most effective, and (b) persons who exhibit flexibility in their efforts are better at coping. In their pioneer work with cancer patients, Weisman and Worden (1976–1977) assessed the use of 15 different types of coping strategies in a sample of 120 newly diagnosed patients. On the basis of clinical interviews and self-report ratings, these authors concluded that the most effective coping strategies involved behaviors that dealt directly and realistically with the illness and related problems. Avoidance, apathy, passivity, and externalizing blame were among the least effective strategies.

STRESS ATTENUATION THROUGH PROBLEM-SOLVING COPING

The second question addresses the issue of whether effective problem solving serves to decrease the likelihood of experiencing distress as a result of encountering a stressful event. Several investigations have provided strong support for a positive answer to this query regarding depression (Kant et al., 1997; A. M. Nezu, Nezu, et al., 1986; A. M. Nezu & Ronan, 1985, 1988) and anxiety (Kant et al., 1997; A. M. Nezu, 1986d). For example, A. M. Nezu, Nezu, et al. (1986) found that among a university student population, problem solving served as a moderator between negative stressful life events and depressive symptoms. Specifically, results from multiple regression analyses indicated that effective problem solvers under high levels of stress reported significantly lower depression scores as compared with ineffective problem solvers under similar levels of high stress. A cross-validation of the regression analysis resulted in a minimal amount of shrinkage that could be due to sample-specific characteristics, thus increasing the validity of these findings. Furthermore, a replication of this study with clinically depressed adults by A. M. Nezu, Perri, Nezu, and Mahoney (1987) provided similar results. Moreover, A. M. Nezu and Ronan (1988), in conducting a prospective study to control for methodological problems potentially associated with cross-sectional analyses, also found strong evidence in support of a moderator effect for problem solving regarding the stress–depression relationship.

A. M. Nezu and Ronan (1985) directly tested the problem-solving model of stress with specific regard to depressive symptomatology. Using path-analytic techniques, they analyzed data from 205 college students to test the following causal relations among these variables: (a) Negative stressful events often result in an increase in problematic situations, (b) degree to which individuals effectively cope with these problems is a function of their problem-solving ability, and (c) effective resolution of these problems decreases the probability of depressive symptoms. In general, results from the path analysis supported this model. They found that negative life stress was associated with depressive symptoms in both a direct fashion and in an indirect manner through increases in the level of current problems. Furthermore, current daily problems had a significant direct impact on depressive symptoms, as well as an indirect influence by the quality of one's problem-solving skills. Finally, problem solving itself had a direct influence on the level of depressive symptoms. This model accounted for over 40% of the variance associated with the prediction of depression scores. These results were later replicated by using a sample of psychiatric patients with a diagnosis of major depressive disorder (A. M. Nezu, Perri, & Nezu, 1987).

To determine whether the same relationships were applicable to cancer-related stress, we conducted a study that included 44 male and 90 female adult cancer patients (A. M. Nezu, Nezu, Faddis, DelliCarpini, & Houts, 1995). Their mean age was close to 50 years, and their diagnoses of cancer were made within the previous 6 months. Over 80% were White, and all were actively undergoing treatment for cancer at the time of the study.

Problem-solving ability was measured by the SPSI–R, whereas distress was defined according to the Depression and Anxiety subscales of the BSI. Cancer-related stress was measured by the CARES, whereby for each cancer-related problem that an individual was experiencing, he or she was also requested to indicate the stressful impact of that problem on a 5-point scale, with responses ranging from 0 (*no problem*) to 4 (*severe problem*). For problem solving to be found to serve as a moderator of the stress–distress relationship, the statistical interactions between problem solving and stress scores need to be significant within a multiple regression analytic approach (Baron & Kenny, 1986). Results indicated that these interactions were significant, thereby suggesting that problem-solving ability does function to moderate the negative effects of cancer-related stress with regard to depressive and anxiety symptoms. More specifically, under similar levels of high cancer-related stress, individuals with poor problem-solving skills reported significantly higher levels of depressive and anxiety symptomatology than individuals characterized by more effective problem-solving skills. Figure 2.2 depicts this relationship with regard to depression.

THE EFFICACY OF PST

The third question relates directly to the issue of the clinical applicability of a problem-solving model of stress and the effectiveness of the associated treatment approach. Problem-solving therapy (PST) has been effective with a wide range of clinical disorders and psychological problems, such as social phobia (DiGiuseppe, Simon, McGowan, &

FIGURE 2.2

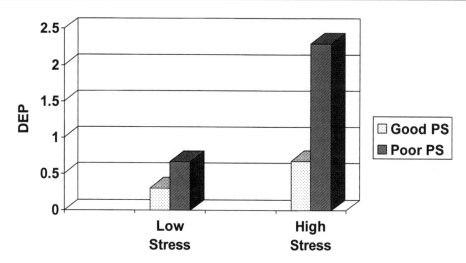

Interaction between cancer-related stress and rational problem-solving skills in predicting depression scores. DEP = depression; PS = problem solving.

Gardner, 1990), agoraphobia (Jannoun, Munby, Catalan, & Gelder, 1980), obesity (Perri, Nezu, & Viegener, 1992), coronary heart disease (Ewart, 1990), schizophrenia (Bradshaw, 1993), mentally retarded adults with concomitant psychiatric problems (C. M. Nezu et al., 1991), HIV risk behaviors (Magura, Kang, & Shapiro, 1994), drug abuse (Platt, Husband, Hermalin, Cater, & Metzger, 1993), suicide (Lerner & Clum, 1990; Salkovkis, Atha, & Storer, 1990), childhood aggression (Pfiffner, Jouriles, Brown, Estcheidt, & Kelly, 1990), and conduct disorder (Kendall & Braswell, 1985).

PST has been found to be effective in particular for clinical depression. For example, Hussian and Lawrence (1981) conducted a study that included depressed older patients to test the relative efficacy of PST and social reinforcement approaches to treatment, as compared with a WLC condition. The superiority of PST over the other two conditions was evident both at posttreatment and at a 2-week follow-up assessment.

A. M. Nezu (1986c) randomly assigned reliably diagnosed depressed adults to one of three conditions: (a) PST, (b) problem-focused therapy (PFT), and (c) WLC. Participants in the PFT group were provided with a similar treatment rationale as that of the PST condition; that is, resolution of problematic situations and other sources of stress would lead to a decrease in depression. However, members of this condition were not provided with a systematic model for problem resolution. Instead, they were encouraged to use the sessions to discuss problems with other group members. Essentially, this treatment condition resembled a group psychotherapy program that emphasized the influence of current difficulties and crises in maintaining or causing depression. It was included as a reasonable treatment alternative providing an appropriate methodological contrast to the PST condition, but it would also be viewed by its members as a legitimate treatment modality. Both treatment programs were conducted over eight 90-minute group sessions.

Results of pre–post analyses indicated that PST participants reported a significant decrease in their depressive symptoms, which was also found to covary with concurrent increases in problem-solving effectiveness and the adoption of an internal locus of control orientation. This improvement was maintained at a 6-month follow-up assessment. Moreover, PST participants reported significantly lower posttreatment depression scores than either the PFT or WLC participants. Further analyses indicated these changes to be clinically meaningful. For example, it was found that 91% of the PST participants showed clinically meaningful improvement, as compared with rates of 22% for PFT participants and 17% for the WLC condition.

As noted earlier, the purpose of a subsequent study by A. M. Nezu and Perri (1989) was to assess the relative contribution of training in the problem orientation component in treating depressed individuals. A dismantling strategy was used to address these goals by randomly assigning adults with diagnoses of major depressive disorder to one of three conditions: (a) PST, (b) abbreviated problem-solving therapy (APST), and (c) WLC. PST participants reported less depressive symptoms at posttreatment, as measured by both a self-report inventory (Beck Depression Inventory; BDI; Beck, Ward, Mendelson, Mock, & Erbaugh, 1961) and a clinician rating (Hamilton Rating Scale for Depression; HRSD; Hamilton, 1960), in comparison to both the APST and WLC participants. Furthermore, APST participants reported significantly lower posttreatment depression scores than WLC participants. Decreases in depressive symptoms were also significantly correlated with increases in problem-solving ability. A 6-month follow-up assessment revealed no significant differences between posttreatment and follow-up scores for either treatment condition. In other words, the therapeutic benefits obtained by participants in both treatment conditions were maintained 6 months after completing treatment. These results suggest that the inclusion of training in problem orientation adds significantly to the overall effectiveness of PST.

Arean et al. (1993) evaluated the efficacy of PST for geriatric depression. Seventy-five older, depressed individuals were randomly assigned to PST, reminiscence therapy (RT), or a WLC condition. Both

PST and RT conditions were conducted within a group format with one of three therapists who were trained in both treatment approaches. Each group met over 12 weekly sessions with each session lasting approximately 1.5 hr. Participants in the PST condition were trained in the five components of problem-solving therapy articulated by A. M. Nezu et al. (1989). RT involved reviewing one's life history to gain perspective and satisfaction with major positive and negative life events and was based on a psychodynamic formulation that had received some empirical support for its efficacy for geriatric depression.

Overall results indicated that participants in the PST and RT therapy conditions were significantly less depressed on three different measures of depression (BDI; HRSD; and Geriatric Depression Scale, Yesavitch et al., 1983) at posttreatment, as compared with WLC individuals. Moreover, the effects found at posttreatment for PST and RT conditions were maintained 3 months after the completion of treatment. Furthermore, individuals in the PST condition reported significantly lower depression at posttreatment than RT participants on two of the three depression measures (i.e., HRSD and GDS). Particularly revealing was the finding that at posttreatment, a significantly greater proportion of individuals in the PST condition (88%), compared with participants in the RT (40%) and WLC (10%) groups, no longer met the diagnostic criteria for major depression.

More recently, Mynors-Wallis, Gath, Lloyd-Thomas, and Tomlinson (1995) compared PST with an antidepressant medication regimen for the treatment of depression in a primary care population. Ninety-one adults with major depression were randomly assigned to PST, amitriptyline, or drug placebo conditions. In all three treatment conditions, participants were offered six or seven sessions lasting from 30 to 60 minutes over 3 months. The three therapists were a psychiatrist and two general practitioners who were trained in PST and drug administration.

In addition to the HRSD, two other outcome measures were used: the BDI and a self-report measure of social functioning and adjustment. Results indicated that at 6 and 12 weeks posttreatment, the PST group was significantly less depressed on both measures of depression and more socially adjusted than the placebo group. No significant differences were found between the PST and amitriptyline conditions. This suggests that for the treatment of depression, PST is as effective as a psychopharmacologic intervention.

PST FOR CANCER PATIENTS

Relevant to this text, interventions that are based on a problem-solving approach have also been applied to cancer patients. For example,

Weisman, Worden, and Sobel (1980) evaluated a problem-solving-based approach for newly diagnosed cancer patients assessed as being at high risk for emotional distress. Two treatment groups that incorporated some training in problem solving were conducted over a 4-week period with a sample of 59 cancer patients. Unfortunately, although significant improvements were demonstrated in terms of lowered emotional distress, the control group against which these conditions were compared involved data collected from a sample from an earlier study. As such, this investigation was not truly randomized and was unable to provide for adequate methodological controls. In addition, from the standpoint of assessing the unique contributions of problem-solving training, the one condition devoted to teaching patients a specific step-by-step problem-solving process also contained instruction in relaxation strategies. Thus, it is difficult to determined if the positive gains associated with this treatment protocol were due to problem solving, relaxation, or placebo.

In fact, although several outcome studies have been conducted since the seminal Weisman et al. (1980) work was published that include some form of problem-solving training as one component of a coping-skills package (e.g., Edgar, Rosberger, & Nowlis, 1992; Fawzy et al., 1990; Telch & Telch, 1986), no study to date has assessed the unique contributions of PST. As such, it is difficult to ascertain whether problem-solving training is a necessary, sufficient, or even effective treatment approach with regard to facilitating adjustment of cancer patients. It is within this context that Project Genesis was developed (A. M. Nezu, Nezu, Friedman, Houts, et al., 1997).

Project Genesis is funded by the National Cancer Institute and represents a large-scale, randomized, prospective outcome study geared to evaluate the effectiveness of PST for adult cancer patients experiencing significant psychological distress. Our major clinical goals are to (a) improve cancer patients' overall problem-solving abilities and skills, (b) decrease their current emotional distress, (c) increase their sense of control by teaching them a set of generalizable coping skills, and (d) improve their overall quality of life. Experimentally, adult cancer patients who meet inclusion and exclusion criteria (e.g., clinically distressed, not receiving therapy from another source, and prognosis of 5-year survival rate of 50% or greater) are randomly assigned to one of three conditions: (a) PST plus standard medical treatment (SMT), (b) PST with significant other plus SMT, and (c) SMT only (WLC). In the PST-plus-SMT condition, patients are taught problem-solving skills in 10 individual 1.5-hr sessions.

In the second treatment condition, patients are taught these skills in tandem with a significant other who functions as a "problem-solving coach." This condition was developed to capitalize on the potential positive effects of formalizing a social support structure. In the SMT-only condition, cancer patients are placed on a waiting list for PST for 10 weeks.

Assessments are conducted pretreatment, posttreatment, 6-months posttreatment, and 1-year posttreatment and include measures of emotional distress, problem solving, locus of control, and cancer-related problems. For ethical purposes, participants in the WLC condition are provided a choice of treatment options after the 10-week waiting period. Thus, there are no follow-up assessment data for WLC participants.

At the time of writing this book, we remain in the data collection and analysis phase. However, initial analyses provide support for the efficacy of PST for distressed cancer patients (A. M. Nezu, Nezu, Friedman, Faddis, & Houts, 1997). When reviewing these results as presented shortly, keep in mind that the data represent preliminary findings and only when the entire data set is completely analyzed will a comprehensive and valid picture emerge. However, the following results are instructive and point to the effectiveness of PST.

The results reported here pertain to comparisons among the first 17 participants in each of the three conditions, who completed either the treatment or the waiting-list period, as well as the 6-month follow-up for the two treatment groups. The mean age of this sample of 34 women and 17 men was approximately 46.5 years. They were diagnosed with cancer within 1 year of their participation in this study. Diagnoses include the following major cancer types: leukemia (28%), breast (41%), urinary (7%), colon (4%), ovarian (4%), cervical (3%) non-Hodgkin'slymphoma (7%), and Hodgkin's disease (6%). Approximately 75% are White, 18% African American, 1% Asian, and 6% Hispanic. Over 76% are married, and collectively they have a mean of 14.79 years of formal education. Although the entire data set contains a variety of measures, we report only the major findings at this time.

Emotional Distress

Measures of psychological distress include the BSI (see earlier description), the Profile of Mood States (POMS; McNair, Lorr, & Droppleman, 1992), and the HRSD. The POMS is a measure of affective states that has frequently been used to assess mood disturbance with cancer patients. The HRSD is a 17-item clinician rating scale for assessing depressive severity that is completed as a function of information gleaned during a semistructured interview. In this study, a number of interviews were randomly selected to include a second interviewer to assess interrater reliability. For these 51 participants, this metric was found to be .87.

In general, results of repeated measures, multivariate analyses of variance (MANOVA) revealed the following: (a) Participants in both treatment conditions, as compared with the WLC, were characterized by significantly lower levels of distress on all three measures at post-treatment; and (b) these positive results were maintained 6 months later. Figure 2.3 depicts these results regarding the HRSD.

To put these results in perspective, consider the "normative" meaning of these scores. Consensus cutoff scores for the HRSD include the following ranges: 25+ indicates severely depressed patients, 18–24 represents the moderate range, 7–17 signifies mild depression, and less than 7 is considered nondepressed (Rabkin & Klein, 1987). The mean across the three conditions at pretreatment was over 19, suggesting that these 51 participants fell in the moderate range of depression. No differences existed regarding depression among the three sets of participants at pretreatment. At posttreatment, however, patients in both treatment conditions were found to be represented with HRSD means of 6.59 (PST) and 7.11 (PST+), whereas WLC participants were rated with a mean of 17.33. These results, therefore, suggest that as a function of undergoing problem-solving therapy, cancer patients became nondepressed and remained so 6 months later. Participants in the WLC condition continued to be moderately depressed.

FIGURE 2.3

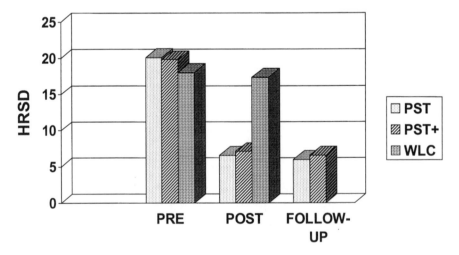

Project Genesis: Hamilton Rating Scale for Depression (HRSD) scores at pretreatment, posttreatment, and 6-month follow-up for first 17 participants in each condition. PST = problem-solving therapy; WLC = waiting-list control.

Cancer-Related Problems

With regard to the CARES, results were similar to the analyses regarding emotional distress, as depicted in Figure 2.4. In other words, both treatment conditions resulted in significant decreases in the number and intensity of cancer-related problems, as compared with the WLC. Furthermore, these results were found to be maintained at the 6-month follow-up assessment point.

To place CARES scores in context, the associated *T* scores, as contained in the CARES manual (Schag & Heinrich, 1989), for the means at pretreatment across the three conditions centered around 72. At posttreatment, the *T* scores for the two treatment conditions were similar and were approximately 51. There was essentially no change in the CARES scores for WLC participants.

Problem Solving

To assess whether PST had an effect on participants' problem-solving ability, we included the SPSI–R as a measure of the mechanism of action. Results of the repeated measures MANOVA indicated that participants in both treatment conditions significantly improved their problem solving from pre- to posttreatment, whereas WLC partici-

FIGURE 2.4

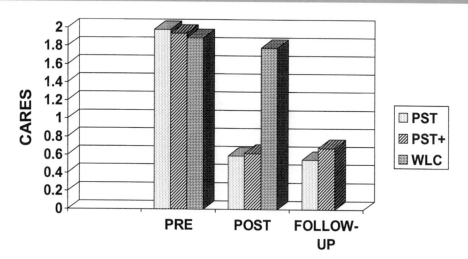

Cancer Rehabilitation Evaluation System (CARES) scores at pretreatment, posttreatment, and 6-month follow-up for first 17 participants in each condition. PST = problem-solving therapy; WLC = waiting-list control.

pants did not. Once again, this positive impact was maintained 6 months later (see Figure 2.5).

Note that the higher the SPSI–R score, the more effective one's problem-solving ability. The mean score total across the three conditions at pretreatment was found to be very similar to the mean included in the SPSI–R manual representing a sample of 74 distressed cancer patients (i.e., cancer patients who were either self- or physician-referred for psychological counseling). At posttreatment, both treatment conditions reported mean SPSI–R total scores more similar to the norms representing a "normal" adult sample. No changes were evident for the WLC participants.

Although these results represent preliminary findings, they collectively underscore the efficacy of PST as a clinical intervention to reduce the emotional distress and to improve the quality of life of patients with cancer. More specifically, with regard to the first 51 participants participating in Project Genesis, PST was found to lead to (a) significant decreases in self-reported and clinician-rated negative affect and depression, (b) significant decreases in cancer-related problems and rehabilitation needs, and (c) significant increases in overall problem-solving ability. These results suggest PST was probably an active and effective component in those studies that included it as one of several treatment elements. As such, PST would appear to be particularly

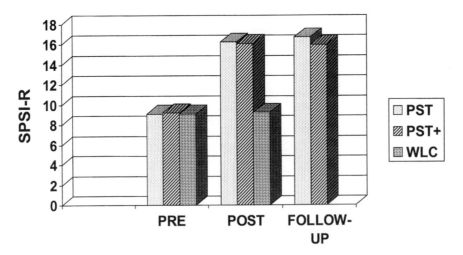

FIGURE 2.5

Project Genesis: Social Problem-Solving Inventory—Revised (SPSI–R) scores at pretreatment, posttreatment, and 6-month follow-up for first 17 participants in each condition. PST = problem-solving therapy; WLC = waiting-list control.

applicable and effective for adult cancer patients experiencing emotional distress and decreased quality of life.

One additional implication of the results from Project Genesis is the lack of an effect related to the inclusion of a significant other in training. Note that with regard to all three assessment domains reported here, no differences between the PST and the PST+ participants were identified. It is possible that involving a patient's significant other as a problem-solving coach is no more effective than training the patient him- or herself. However, because of the impressive results obtained thus far, a floor or ceiling effect may have occurred. In other words, PST alone leads to maximal effects, in which adding another potentially efficacious intervention component cannot demonstrate additional benefits beyond that already achieved. Future research may need to address this question more systematically. At this stage, however, if asked for our clinical opinion regarding whether to include a significant other in treatment, on the basis of the present findings, we would suggest that if both individuals agree, then it may be beneficial. Conversely, if the cancer patient prefers not to include a family member or friend, then this request should be respected (see also chapter 3).

Summary and Conclusions

This chapter began with several definitions related to problem solving. More specifically, *problem solving* was described as the process by which individuals understand the nature of problems in living and direct their coping efforts at altering the problematic nature of the situations themselves, their reactions to them, or both. *Problems* were defined as specific life circumstances that demand responses for adaptive functioning but were not met with effective coping responses from the individuals confronted with them because of the presence of various obstacles. *Effective solutions* are those coping responses that not only achieve such goals but also simultaneously maximize other positive consequences and minimize other negative consequences.

In addition, we described effective problem solving as comprising five interacting component processes, each of which makes a distinct contribution to effective problem resolution. These include *problem orientation, problem definition* and *formulation, generation of alternatives, decision making*, and *solution implementation* and *verification*.

The relevance of problem-solving coping to cancer-related distress was delineated within the context of a problem-solving model of stress, which was portrayed as a dynamic function of the reciprocal relationships among major negative life events, daily problems, negative emotional states, and problem-solving coping. Cancer and the related medical and psychosocial problems that it engenders were conceptualized as major sources of stress that can greatly affect one's quality of life negatively. More important, the more effective persons are in resolving or coping with such illness-related difficulties, the more probable it is that they will not experience significant distress. Conversely, if a cancer patient has difficulty in coping with such problems, he or she will likely experience depression, anxiety, and other distress symptoms.

Three research questions were posed to assess the validity and applicability of this model to cancer. They include the following: (a) Is there a significant inverse relationship between problem solving and psychological distress? (b) Does effective problem-solving skills attenuate distress engendered by stressful events? and (c) Does therapeutic interventions that are based on problem-solving training lead to meaningful reductions in distress?

Findings from a variety of studies were provided that support the validity of the model in general, as well as its applicability to cancer patients. With regard to PST itself, several studies focused on depression were briefly highlighted to underscore its overall efficacy. Moreover, we described Project Genesis, a large-scale, prospective outcome investigation that is geared to assess the effectiveness of PST for cancer patients. Preliminary findings from this project were offered that strongly indicate that PST is a potent intervention to help improve the quality of life of cancer patients.

The remainder of this book provides for a detailed description of how to implement PST for distressed cancer patients. The next chapter specifically addresses general characteristics of this approach, whereas the remaining chapters provide for a detailed "treatment manual."

II | AN OVERVIEW OF TRAINING

Problem-Solving Therapy for Cancer Patients:

Overview, Process, and Related Clinical Issues

3

Overview

I
n this section of the book, we present a detailed therapy manual that provides specific guidelines in conducting problem-solving therapy (PST) for cancer patients. In the present chapter, we discuss various general clinical issues, such as the structure of problem-solving therapy, assessment guidelines, the therapist–patient relationship, and the use of adjunctive therapeutic strategies.

What Is PST for Cancer Patients?

PST encompasses a collection of strategies aimed at helping individuals to understand the nature of problems in living and directs their attempts at changing the nature of the problematic situation itself, their reactions to them, or both. PST for cancer patients is especially focused toward psychosocial problems related to cancer and its treatment. As with other applications of PST, this one emphasizes (a) a collaborative relationship between patient and therapist; (b) an ongoing assessment of progress (or lack of progress); (c) the goal of increasing skill competencies regarding specific cognitive, affective, and behavioral targets, including planned strategies for maintenance; and (d) the prevention of future symptoms of distress. However, the adaptation of PST to cancer patients additionally emphasizes attention to the cumulative physical, social, and psychological stressors present for such individuals. Finally, although patients with cancer might be viewed as medically homogeneous, it is important to recognize that their psychological histories are extremely diverse. Flexibility is inherent in a problem-solving approach. This increases the applicability of the intervention to a broad range of individuals. As such, PST may be helpful for a woman in midlife who has undergone a mastectomy and experiencing fear and avoidance of sexual intimacy, as well as for a young adult man with leukemia who is experiencing family difficulties concerning his independence.

PST Treatment Goals

Overall, the goals of PST are to help distressed cancer patients to (a) identify previous and current life situations (i.e., major life events such as cancer diagnosis and treatment, as well as current daily problems associated with such events) that serve to increase the intensity and frequency of their distress; (b) reduce the extent to which distressful emotions, such as anxiety, anger, and depressive symptoms, negatively affect their current and future attempts at coping; (c) increase the effectiveness of their problem-solving coping attempts concerning current problem situations; and (d) teach skills that will enable them to deal more effectively with future problems to prevent severe or debilitating negative emotional reactions.

As indicated previously (see also chapter 2), depending on the patients' particular life circumstances and characteristics of both their medical and psychological treatment, PST can focus on helping patients to change the problematic nature of the situation (e.g., less physical energy), the negative emotional responses to the situation (e.g., reducing fear of computerized tomography scan), or both (e.g., difficulty making medical treatment decisions). In most clinical cases, addressing both aspects is usually advisable and important. For example, problems with making medical treatment decisions frequently involve difficulties associated with the situation, such as lack of medical information. In addition, such problems can also involve difficulties stemming from one's own psychological, emotional, or philosophical responses. Examples of these may include fears that impede logical thinking, avoidance, anger over the burden of the diagnoses, or spiritual beliefs surrounding healing or death.

When Is PST Appropriate for Cancer Patients?

Because PST is based on a skills competency model of intervention, this form of psychosocial therapy can be viewed as useful to any individual undergoing cancer treatment and at almost any point in medical treatment. This begins with the time before diagnosis, when worries and fears are rampant because of a suspicious mole, bleeding, persistent cough, or significant family history. The plethora of problems experienced as a function of the diagnosis and treatment was discussed in detail in chapter 1—all of these problems provide possible points of entry to psychological treatment for the person with cancer. All of the various problems described in chapter 1 in the *Pathways of Patients' Psychological Experience* section can provide further impetus for seeking or being referred for psychological intervention. Last, even after active medical treatment, because of fears of recurrence, changing relationships and family roles, and sometimes existential questions and insights following their experience, cancer patients might pursue psychological treatment.

To date, there is little empirical evidence to help determine whether various cancer patient characteristics or circumstances exist that relate to treatment success or failure. Clinical experience does suggest that as a major treatment modality, PST is appropriate for a wide range of psychological and psychiatric referral symptoms and for a wide range of nonpsychotic mood disorders, especially major depression. Patients who have participated within our research programs span a wide range of ages, socioeconomic status, educational levels, ethnic backgrounds, history of previous episodes of anxiety and depression, and psychotherapy contacts. As such, applying PST on an individual or group basis can be very effective. To facilitate this process, the unique history and personal learning experiences that a person brings to treatment should meaningfully be incorporated into the overall intervention plan.

The presence of severe melancholia, psychotic symptomatology, advanced dementing illnesses, or significant cognitive limitations that are due to a brain metastasis may be contraindicative of this approach. On the other hand, individuals with a history of psychotic illness who are well stabilized through appropriate medication, as well as individuals with mild cognitive or intellectual impairment, need not be ruled out as viable candidates for PST. In such cases, providing explanations and using training materials with clear and concrete language, more visual examples, interactive strategies, and greater repetition can produce impressive results with such patients. As noted in chapter 2, for example, PST has been shown to be effective in reducing psychological distress and in improving adaptive functioning of adults with limited cognitive abilities (i.e., mental retardation; C. M. Nezu et al., 1991).

Persons exhibiting significant characterological disturbance, such as borderline personality features or individuals with a history of substance abuse, may require adjunctive treatments that initially provide greater external structure and support. In such cases, PST can be combined with other approaches in a strategic and integrated manner. For example, patients with substance abuse histories may require medication or additional group or individual treatments that specifically address the substance abuse problem. Patients with personality disorders may benefit from PST conducted in a group format, with individual sessions that monitor progress and focus on additional emotional-regulation training. The group milieu can provide a "safe" environment in which to practice new problem-solving skills in interpersonal situations that can be particularly difficult for such individuals.

The Process of PST

In general, PST, similar to other psychotherapies, can conceptually be divided into three major stages: (a) assessment, (b) treatment, and (c) maintenance and generalization training.

ASSESSMENT

Assessment of Distress

One of the most important ways to gather initial information concerning differential diagnosis, as well as the prevalence and extent of current patient difficulties, is through a semistructured interview. Especially if conducted as part of individual therapy, the interview is a critical time to create an atmosphere of trust and open communication that can continue throughout treatment. Knowledge of the current *Diagnostic and Statistical Manual of Mental Disorders* (DSM–IV; American Psychiatric Association, 1994) is important and useful with regard to conducting a differential diagnosis. However, in addition to collecting information about a patient's current and specific diagnostic symptoms, it is necessary to gather a comprehensive history including data about past diagnoses, outpatient treatments and hospitalizations, current cancer treatment, complications, decisions, course of chemotherapy and radiation, current prescription and nonprescription drug usage, educational, social, family background, spiritual–philosophical beliefs, and current level of functioning. Important are inquiries about the patient's use of alcohol and other substances and potential for suicide. If a strong indication of suicide potential is present, then further inquiries concerning whether the patient has an active suicidal plan is essential. As an adjunct to PST "proper," crisis intervention and close moment-by-moment monitoring may be necessary during times of active suicidal thoughts, especially when any substance use may be involved.

In addition to interview assessment, a variety of self-report measures should be administered to obtain vital information about the patient. However, it is important to recognize that persons undergoing cancer treatment may easily be distracted and experience extreme fatigue. Therefore, the clinician needs to be sensitive regarding the amount of paper-and-pencil measures that will be required early in treatment.

One self-report measure is the Brief Symptom Inventory (BSI; Derogatis & Spencer, 1982), which provides for a quantitative evaluation of distress. As indicated in chapter 2, the BSI is a 53-item self-report measure of psychological distress symptoms experienced by both medical and psychiatric patients. Each item is rated on a 5-point scale of distress, with responses ranging from 0 (*not at all*) to 4 (*extremely*). The BSI has been used in several studies that have assessed the prevalence of psychopathology in cancer populations and has been shown to be a particularly valid and useful measure for psychosocial screening of newly diagnosed cancer patients (Zabora et al., 1990). The BSI can be scored for nine primary symptom dimensions (i.e., somatization, obsessive–compulsive, interpersonal sensitivity, depression, anxiety, hostility, phobic anxiety, paranoid ideation, and psychoticism). The Depression and Anxiety subscales are of particular interest to many clinicians working with persons diagnosed with cancer because they represent the more typical psychosocial reactions to stressful events. The Depression subscale reflects various aspects of clinical depression (e.g., feelings of hopelessness and dysphoric mood), whereas the Anxiety subscale addresses symptoms associated with manifest anxiety (e.g., feeling fearful and signs of nervous tension). In general, the BSI is characterized by strong internal consistency and test–retest reliability properties.

Other measures of anxiety and depression with which a clinician may be familiar, such as the various Minnesota Multiphasic Personality Inventory subscales (Dahlstrom & Welsh, 1960), the Beck Depression Inventory (Beck et al., 1961), the Hamilton Rating Scale for Depression (Hamilton, 1967), and the State–Trait Anxiety

Inventory (Spielberger, Gorsuch, & Lushene, 1979), can also be used to more carefully pinpoint symptoms or patient complaints.

Assessment of Quality of Life

As indicated in chapter 2, the Cancer Evaluation and Rehabilitation Evaluation System (CARES; Schag & Heinrich, 1989) was designed to assess day-to-day problems and rehabilitation needs of cancer patients. It is a revision of the earlier Cancer Inventory of Problem Situations Inventory (Schag, Heinrich, & Ganz, 1983) that was developed using a competency-based model of coping as its theoretical underpinning (see Goldfried & D'Zurilla, 1969). Patients rate each problem on a 5-point scale, with responses ranging from 0 (*no problem*) to 4 (*severe problem*). Various forms exist for clinical and research purposes. In Project Genesis (see chapter 2), we use the research version that contains 59 items and that can be scored to obtain a global score, as well as the following five scale scores: physical, psychosocial, medical interaction, marital, and sexual problems. These scales were derived on the basis of item reduction and factor-analytic techniques.

The CARES has been normed on a sample of over 1,000 cancer patients and has been found to possess strong psychometric properties of reliability and validity (Schag et al., 1990). For example, test–retest estimates of the total score and the five major scales range between .84 and .91. The CARES provides for a comprehensive list of problems encountered by cancer patients as they cope with the disease and its treatment on a regular basis.

Another quality-of-life measure is the Functional Assessment of Cancer Therapy (FACT) Scale. The FACT is a brief, yet sensitive, 33-item quality-of-life measure for evaluating patients receiving cancer treatment. The FACT is useful in clinical research trials because it is easy to administer and is brief, reliable, valid, and responsive to clinical change (Cella et al., 1993). Coefficients of reliability and validity are uniformly high. A 28-item version of the measure that was the product of factor-analytic studies provides subscale scores in addition to the total score for physical, functional, social, and emotional well-being. In addition, there is a variety of versions geared to assess specific cancer types (e.g., prostate, breast, and lung), treatment approaches (e.g., bone marrow transplant and biologic response modifiers), and specific symptoms (e.g., fatigue and anemia).

Another quality-of-life measure is the Quality-of-Life Index (Spitzer et al., 1981), which measures the general well-being of patients who are terminally ill with cancer or other chronic diseases. It is a brief instrument to evaluate the effects of treatment and programs such as palliative care, but it has subsequently been used more broadly (McDowell & Newell, 1996). The SF-36, or Short Form–36 Health Survey (Ware & Sherbourne, 1992), was designed as a generic indicator of health status for use in population surveys and evaluative studies of health policy. It is usually used in conjunction with disease-specific measures to assess outcome in research and clinical practice.

A final measure is the Functional Living Index—Cancer (Schipper, Clinch, McMurray, & Levitt, 1984). This scale was developed to determine the response of cancer patients to their diagnoses, illness experience, and treatment. It was proposed as an adjunct to clinical assessments of progress in clinical research trials.

Several additional inventories exist that provide information concerning types of recently experienced stressful events. Checklists such as the Mooney Problem Checklist (Mooney & Gordon, 1950) or the Personal Problems Checklist (Schinka, 1986) are useful to assess additional non-cancer-related problems that may have served as minor stressful events.

Assessment of Problem Solving

To provide individualized treatment, the therapist should conduct a comprehensive assessment of the patient's current level of problem-solving functioning during the initial interviews. It is important to observe and analyze what coping attempts the patient has previously tried for dealing with cancer-related problems. Such questions should be couched in terms of information gathering with a view to minimize the possibility that the patient perceives them as criticisms about their poor coping ability. Interview assessment should entail inquiries regarding all facets of the problem-solving model, including a patient's initial perceptions of the event, how goals were defined, what actual alternatives were considered, whether he or she actually implemented any solutions, and how the patient felt about the outcome.

CASE EXAMPLE

Clinical Case: Rob

The following is an example of the beginning of such an interview with a patient named Rob after a consultation request from his oncologist. After undergoing a successful bone marrow transplant, Rob indicated to his doctor that he was extremely depressed and suicidal. He reported to the problem-solving therapist that he had left his wife after 5 years of an unsatisfactory marriage, but his decision was not receiving the support he had hoped it would from his family.

THERAPIST. What have you tried to do to improve this situation, Rob?

ROB. I tried to explain to my family that I can't live a lie anymore, not after everything I've been through—but they don't understand. In fact, my dad thinks the chemo has affected my brain and changed my personality. Don't they realize that I'm not the same person I was before? I've been through more problems than most people who are my age! I get so angry at people sometimes that I don't know what to do.

THERAPIST. So you're feeling pretty helpless about solving this problem. You want your family's support in this decision, but you don't have it.

ROB. I can't. They'll never change. No matter what I do or say. I didn't mean to scare my doctor when I said I wanted to kill myself. I wouldn't really do it, but I felt like it.

THERAPIST. What have you tried to do about the problem with your family?

ROB. Talk to them. What else is there? But I get so angry, I end up yelling. That just makes them think that I am crazy and out of control.

THERAPIST. There may be other alternative ways to work on this problem.

ROB. I don't know. I mean if they can't understand that I need to make these changes in my life . . . forget it, forget them . . . I don't even want to think about it.

THERAPIST. And it sounds like all of this has become such a burden, because the one solution you came up with didn't work out at all the way you expected or hoped. Let me see if I can summarize part of what is happening to you now. You find yourself actually facing additional problems, like doing something for the first time that is for your own approval, rather than your family's approval or someone else's wishes.

ROB. I'm sick of living my life for other people—I just want some happiness for myself—I don't know how long I will be around.

THERAPIST. This change in the way you view others and your desire to behave in a different way than you have in the past is a problem in and of itself.

ROB. You think there's something else I can do here?

THERAPIST.   I know there are other things you can do. There are specific strategies to understanding emotions and solving problems that you can learn that are likely to improve the situation for you. You notice that I said improve, rather than remove, the problematic situation. That's because the way you look at problems and the expectations that you have can also affect your ability to cope.

Clinical Commentary

Early in this assessment, specific deficits appear to be emerging. There is an orientation that is focused on expectations of correct and immediate solutions, as well as a minimal degree of tolerance for distress and disappointment. In addition, Rob has an impulsive emotional style that is evident in the way he tends to jump on the first solution that comes to mind. Finally, this patient seems to have "defined himself" in the past on the basis of the expectations of others. On the other hand, Rob reveals some strengths. Despite an impulsive and dramatic communication style observed in his suicidal statements, he acknowledges that his emotions at the time were associated with such comments, that he can inhibit the impulse to act on such extreme thoughts, and he possesses a willingness to discuss his difficulties in a collaborative manner with a therapist.

In addition to interview material that focuses on current life problems and coping attempts, administration of the Social Problem Solving Inventory—Revised (SPSI–R) can provide for both a molar and a molecular evaluation of one's problem-solving ability. That is, in addition to an overall assessment of one's problem-solving processes, the subscales of the SPSI–R provide for a discriminative assessment of the various problem-solving components.

The SPSI–R is a 52-item self-report instrument developed by D'Zurilla et al. (in press) that is linked to the five-dimensional model of social problem-solving described in chapter 2. The subscales were derived from a factor-analytic study (Maydeu-Olivares & D'Zurilla, 1996), which was based on the original 70-item Social Problem-Solving Inventory (D'Zurilla & Nezu, 1990). The SPSI–R measures two constructive problem-solving dimensions (i.e., positive problem orientation and rational problem solving) and three dysfunctional dimensions (i.e., negative problem orientation, impulsivity–carelessness style, and avoidance style). Psychometrically, the SPSI–R is characterized by strong reliability and validity estimates. As such, the SPSI–R provides an extremely important tool for social problem-solving research and clinical assessment.

In the example provided above, Rob's scores on the SPSI–R revealed that he had both a negative problem orientation and an impulsive–carelessness style of attempting to solve problems. Regarding his rational problem-solving skills, he revealed significant deficits in his ability to generate creative solutions, and he experienced difficulty when attempting to define a problem. Using the interview material, combined with his SPSI–R scores, the therapist was able to identify specific deficits in problem-solving component skills as important treatment targets for Rob.

Assessment of Coping Attempts

In keeping with the philosophy of continuous monitoring and evaluation, various assessment measures can also be administered throughout the course of treatment. In addition to the various homework assignments, these include periodic reevaluations of relevant distress measures such as the BSI and the *Record of Coping Attempts* handout (see Figure 3.1). This recording form has space for individuals to (a) provide a written description of a recently experienced problem situation; (b) list thoughts, feelings, and coping behavior within the situation; and (c) rate their overall satisfaction with their coping response. This record can be administered at pretreatment as an assessment strategy, as well as being frequently assigned during the first few sessions to provide important clinical information concerning the relevant problems and areas of coping vulnerabilities for each individual patient. The record of coping attempts should be considered an essential assessment tool and a means of identifying relevant current problems and individual patient coping styles.

INTERVENTION

PST itself focuses primarily on training patients in the five major component problem-solving processes (i.e., problem orientation, problem definition and formulation, generation of alternatives, decision making, and solution implementation and verification). In the remaining chapters, we provide a detailed description of how to implement this intervention protocol. In addition, however, we recommend the use of various adjunctive training strategies and therapy techniques to enhance effective learning and skill acquisition. More specifically, we advocate actively using the following therapeutic strategies when implementing PST: instruction, handouts, teaching metaphors, prompting, modeling, behavioral rehearsal, homework assignments, shaping, reinforcement, and feedback.

FIGURE 3.1

RECORD OF COPING ATTEMPTS

Description of problem situation:

Thoughts (before, during, and after the situation):

Feelings (before, during, and after the situation):

Actual coping behavior:

How pleased were you with your general reaction to the problem? (circle one)

1	2	3	4	5
Not at all		Somewhat		Very Much

Record of coping attempts.

Instruction is an inherent aspect in presenting each new skill. The rationale of each component skill should be presented with special care. Often misapplication of a problem-solving skill area may be caused by the therapist's inattention to the need for providing the information to the patient in a clear, concise, and understandable manner. This material can be presented *didactically* (e.g., using teaching metaphors and relevant examples), as well as in the form of *handouts*. In either format, it is important to use language that is concrete and unambiguous, in keeping with the philosophy of the approach, as well as on the reading level of a particular patient population.

As will become evident throughout this book, we have developed many handouts that supplement the didactic instructions. We have attempted to make these handouts user friendly, attractive, engaging, as well as informative. We strongly recommend the use of such handouts to facilitate the entire skill acquisition and learning process. In addition, we believe that providing patients with three-ring binders, in which they can keep these handouts, serves to increase adherence and foster homework completion. Patients have rated this component very highly in terms of aspects of the treatment that have been particularly helpful. In many ways, having their "own problem-solving book" has served to enhance motivation. Furthermore, they are able to refer to this material in the future if necessary without having to seek formal therapy.

We also use the technique of the *teaching metaphor* throughout PST. The use of a simple picture, story, or parable can often capture a sophisticated and complex metacognitive concept. One example involves the image of a survivor "climbing the stairs" from a victim to survivor during problem orientation training (see chapter 5, Figure 5.2). In this case, the story facilitates a patient's insight regarding the complex interplay of cognitive, affective, and behavioral response styles that are important to successful survival.

Prompting is a procedure in which a cue is provided that helps lead an individual to a correct response. The problem-solving therapist should offer continuous prompts during training in the specific problem-solving skills. For example, a prompt during brainstorming sessions may require the therapist to begin generating alternative solutions. This helps facilitate the patient's skill acquisition. Prompts can also be particularly useful when discussing potential consequences of various decisions or alternative solutions during the decision-making phase.

Shaping is the process by which a response is gradually changed in quality. As such, it is useful to generate a hierarchy of a patient's problems, on the basis of the dimensions of severity and complexity. Less complicated problems can be used in early stages of training as examples of various skills to maximize the chance of initial successful results. As the patients become more confident in their problem-solving ability, the skills can be applied to more difficult and complex problems.

Modeling is a very powerful and important teaching procedure. Within this treatment approach, modeling by the therapist of all problem-solving operations is important. This can be done in vivo or through films, videotapes, or role playing. In addition to modeling applications of PST during sessions, it can be very useful to have the patients observe the behavior of people they see as competent and effective in their own environment outside of session. To facilitate learning and to help individuals discriminate more effectively, it is important to model both efficacious and ineffective ways to apply problem-solving skills. Conducting PST in a group format provides for a particularly powerful use of the strategy.

Behavioral rehearsal or practice of the various problem-solving operations is extremely important in order to maximize skill acquisition. Various analogies about learning any new skill more effectively, such as a new medical self-care regimen, driving a car, or learning a foreign language, take practice. For example, the following statement highlights the importance of practice:

> Remember when you first began learning how to drive a car. The various dials on the dashboard were difficult to understand. The wheel seemed awkward. You were not sure when to put your foot on the brake. You may have felt scared and uncomfortable. How much should I turn the wheel when I make a turn? When should I put the turn signals on? How do I pull out on the highway? These may have been questions you initially asked yourself when you first tried to drive. Now you drive almost everyday of your life. You no longer ask these questions because driving has become a habit. But now what if you drive in a new and confusing place—like a foreign country? Or, you are in very busy traffic or in bad weather? Some new questions and old fears about driving reemerge until you figure out how to manage all of this new information. You may have to back up and go slowly; maybe learn some additional skills. This is what you are doing with all of the new information, problems, and emotions associated with cancer. Slowing down your thoughts and feelings, taking your time to learn some new skills.

Practice or rehearsal should occur both during sessions and between them. As a means of facilitating extra session practice, *homework assignments* are an important feature of the treatment approach. It is clinically useful to characterize the importance of homework by pointing out that a 1- or 2-hour session amounts to only 1/168th or

1/84th of a week's time. To have a major impact on real-life situations, PST needs to be continued by patients on their own between sessions.

Homework assignments can be given at the end of each session and usually correspond to a particular problem-solving operation that was discussed during the session. In the later sessions, more emphasis is given to applying the entire model to real-life situations. Such in vivo applications are an especially important component of the intervention. There are examples of homework sheets that are provided in chapters 5–9 and that correspond to each component skill training.

The problem-solving therapist should also provide *reinforcement* to patients for any and all attempts to engage in the problem-solving process. Therapist reinforcement is an extremely powerful means of increasing patient attempts at problem solving. Reinforcement is part of a larger *feedback* approach that should be incorporated throughout treatment. Reinforcement and feedback should be provided with regard to several important and specific areas—attempts to engage in problem solving, all attempts to complete homework (regardless of quality), any improvement in correct application over previous performance, successful emotional regulation and problem-solving attitude or orientation, and any questions or probes on the patients' part to better understand or learn more about problem solving.

GENERALIZATION AND MAINTENANCE TRAINING

Practice is viewed as an inherent part of PST geared to facilitate maintenance and generalization. Because the overall thrust of this approach is to train people in skills that will contribute to self-control, self-efficacy, and self-regulation, a fair degree of relapse prevention is built into the active treatment component. However, as noted previously, substantial practice in these skills is extremely important. Therefore, maintenance is enhanced if patients are helped and encouraged to apply the entire model across a wide range of problematic situations. For each new problematic situation addressed, patients are encouraged to go through all five major training components as a means of practice. This is why sessions specifically devoted to practice are included in the recommended protocol. In addition, even if patients believe that such a progression is not necessary, it provides the therapist with an assessment of how patients are applying the problem-solving components to their life. When therapy is ending, PST skills can strategically be directed toward working through problems that predictably emerge in the therapy termination process.

Therapist Variables

As a general strategy, it is important for the problem-solving therapist to display warmth, empathy, trust, and a sense of genuineness (Rogers, 1957; Truax & Carkhuff, 1967). However, these characteristics represent minimally required, but not sufficient, skill areas. Because a therapist is changing what may be long-term patterns of reacting to stress, including tendencies to react impulsively, engage in cognitive distortions, and subsequent avoidance reactions, patients may begin to perceive a therapist's attempts to help them change as an attack on their style or personality. It is essential that therapists communicate an acceptance and respect for the individual while simultaneously explaining why certain thinking and reaction habits or patterns may actually be working against the patients' goals.

The therapists must also realize that when attempting to change well-learned behavior, most people will experience a degree of fear, frustration, and anger. These reactions are often directed toward the therapist. Practicing the philosophy of PST, the therapist's objectivity in observing, understanding, and analyzing these reactions will guide him or her toward the appropriate therapeutic solution. For example, one patient with prostate cancer, John, had a history of a domineering and aggressive style. Lacking "psychological sophistication," he frequently changed appointments, made unrealistic demands, and behaved in a rude manner with his female therapist. Rather than react to his attacks personally, his therapist allowed her own anger toward the patient to occur, but pass. She knew that her own reaction signaled the need that she should observe his behavior and attempt to understand what function it served for John. She was able to view John's "therapy battles" within the context of his attempts to cope with a profound sense of loss of control and masculinity. His poor problem solving led him to attempt to improve his sense of control at any given moment by "winning" these perceived battles with his therapist. In John's case, his therapist's validation of his anger over both real and perceived losses, and the use of a metaphor that John was "picking up a sword to attack" when he felt as though he was not in control, were useful interventions. Finally, the therapist urged John to frame PST as not something that belonged to her but something that could be useful and important to him. This served to increase his willingness to learn the skills.

It is important for the problem-solving therapist to be well versed in the areas of depression, anxiety, stress, coping, social problem solving, and in the medical aspects and the predictable course of cancer treatment. A reasonable amount of preparation and understanding of the illness is required to convey to the cancer patient a sense of expertise and competence.

In addition, the best therapists for this approach are the ones who tend to use problem-solving strategies in their own life as a means of coping with stressful situations. This is especially valid if the stressful situation actually involves conducting PST for the first time. For example, we have frequently observed beginning therapists (e.g., psychology students, interns, psychiatric residents, and nurse practitioners) frequently demonstrate a predictable naivete in their initial approach to training in certain problem orientation variables. Armed with a plethora of information concerning the types of selective thinking processes and negative appraisals and attributions often associated with disorders such as depression and anxiety, student therapists often report surprise and frustration when patients resist changing these beliefs. They wonder why their patients are so stubborn or resistive. These students, however, are often wrestling with their own self-evaluations of competency and desire to be helpful and successful. Use of the PST perspective allows novice therapists to see how these fears are predictable problems in their own training "that need to be solved."

Finally, the best problem-solving therapist is one who also uses these strategies and principles as a guide in his or her clinical decision making and judgment. We have presented a comprehensive model of clinical decision making on the basis of a problem-solving formulation elsewhere (A. M. Nezu & Nezu, 1989; A. M. Nezu, Nezu, Friedman, & Haynes, 1997). In essence, this model posits that a therapist needs to be flexible when thinking about developing individualized patient programs and being aware of various errors and biases inherent in human judgment. Use of the various problem-solving operations, such as brainstorming a comprehensive list of treatment strategies for a given patient with a given set of symptoms, increases the likelihood that treatment will be effective.

The Therapist–Patient Relationship

As in other forms of psychotherapy, the therapist–patient relationship is also important to a problem-solving approach. Although PST consists of various training modules, minimization of the therapist–patient relationship can have a severe impact on the overall effectiveness of treatment. Particularly when patients hold beliefs that result in fears of independent functioning and competency, there may exist a strong resistance to learn strategies that would increase self-efficacy and that would help individuals to function more independently. There may be less anxiety, initially, for such individuals to engage in a counseling approach that relies more on the therapist's problem-solving abilities and that provides patients with a strong sense of social support. We have found it useful to have the therapist call patients a short time prior to their scheduled appointment to confirm arrangements and to answer any concerns that are likely to influence their attendance. The approach that we believe communicates the most respect for patients is one in which the therapist approaches the case with confidence as a scientist to observe, question, test, and synthesize information, and not "to fix everything."

In addition, the therapist should attempt to strike a meaningful balance between being an active and directive practitioner and conveying a sense of collaboration with the patient. Because of the inherent psychoeducational flavor of PST, we often present the role of problem-solving therapist as a "teacher." Moreover, analogies such as becoming a team of "investigative reporters," "detectives," or "personal scientists" are often useful in characterizing this collaborative relationship between the therapist and the patient. In other words, these analogies help convey (a) a sense of mutual exploration into the nature of a patient's problems and experience of cancer-related distress and (b) the framework of being active members of a team working toward a mutual goal of "getting at the bottom of the story," "solving a mystery," or "testing certain scientific hypotheses."

Problem Solving Therapy
Do's and Don'ts

In this next section, we offer a discussion of PST "Do's and Don'ts" to foster the recognition for a balanced professional, empathic, and insightful view of the overall therapy process. Moreover, regardless of how effective a given therapy approach has been shown to be, the actual implementation of the treatment can be fraught with problems. Each "do and don't" is followed by an explanation and advice as to how best avoid this potential problem area.

1. DO: Incorporate PST into a patient's overall treatment plan and reason for seeking treatment.
   DON'T: View PST as only skills training and not psychotherapy.

Training in PST presumes an understanding of basic psycho-therapy and counseling skills and focuses on ways in which to provide a patient with a new competency in several important and structured content areas. However, the therapist seeks to increase the individual's skills within the context of a positive and collaborative relationship. Furthermore, the therapist should attempt to evaluate how these skills may best be uniquely understood, learned, and ultimately incorporated into the life of each patient.

2. DO: Work PST into each patient's unique treatment experience and each therapist's unique counseling style.
   DON'T: Present training in a mechanistic manner.

Problems with chronic illness are wrought with distressful and overwhelming emotions. One of the most challenging tasks facing a therapist who is working with people diagnosed with cancer and other chronic illnesses is to help them believe that the way a person thinks can actually combat negative emotions and improve functioning. This requires continual assessment of how the training specifically and relevantly applies to each particular patient at each point in the therapy process. Furthermore, the therapist should be continually aware of what is happening moment by moment in the therapy relationship itself. A patient who believes that his or her goal for coming to therapy is not being addressed, or that the therapist is too much of a "lecturer" and not enough of a "listener," is likely to drop out of treatment.

3. DO: Consistently demonstrate respect for the patient's feelings and foster the notion that he or she can use these negative emotions as important information (i.e., that a problem exists).
   DON'T: Focus only on specific skills training and not on the patient's feelings.

This "Don't" is a sure way to sabotage the treatment process from the beginning. Negative emotions, such as fear, anger, and sadness, are disabling and troublesome experiences that can halt rational thinking. Helping a patient to see that such emotions can actually serve a purpose and direct him or her toward ways in which the patient can improve his or her quality of life is difficult, but important. The therapist who is confronted with such intense feelings of distress will have to examine his or her own comfort with such distress and be prepared to work collaboratively with the patient in managing and regulating these feelings. As emotions emerge during various training sequences, they should be recognized, acknowledged, "validated," and used as an important part of the patient's learning experience. Attempting to focus treatment away from feelings, and trying to enforce training in specific skills without the focus on emotion, is likely to be ineffective and potentially harmful to the patient.

4. DO: Ensure that therapy is made relevant to a given patient.
   DON'T: Deliver a "canned" treatment that does not incorporate relevant life experiences of a given patient.

Consistent with a cognitive approach to treatment, a person's thoughts will affect his or her emotions. As such, initial thoughts or views of PST will affect an individual's initial emotional response to the treatment itself. It is therefore important to use relevant examples of a person's life to communicate concepts. Because there are instances in everyone's life in which it can be shown that objective, flexible thinking can be helpful, even in times of crisis and upheaval, the therapist can usually draw from whatever daily activities, professions, hobbies, or work that an individual typical engages in to develop specific and relevant examples. It is also important to develop an expectancy of what this training can offer at present, when so many resources of time and effort need to be directed to medical care. It is important for the patient to perceive such training as important and helpful for his or her psychological and emotional strength.

5. DO: Incorporate homework into the treatment, reinforce the patient's attempts to complete the homework, and always follow up and attend to all possible homework assignments.
   DON'T: Forget to incorporate homework into treatment.

No treatment works when isolated from a person's everyday life. The danger of not incorporating homework into treatment is that the best outcome possible is one in which the patient views the therapist as a caring problem solver but who never learns to use PST instrumentally for him- or herself.

6. DO: Use humor judiciously.
   DON'T: Assume that the patient will always benefit from the use of humor.

Humor can be helpful when it provides an opportunity for a therapist and a patient to experience a shared insight or gain some cognitive distance from the problem by looking at it differently. In fact, research has indicated that a good sense of humor actually serves to moderate the negative effects of stress (A. M. Nezu, Nezu, & Blissett, 1988). Furthermore, Greenwald (1975) suggested that when a therapist's humor is based on an appreciation of a patient's strengths and abilities, the use of humor can provide a powerful message of belief in the patient's ability to get past his or her suffering and to learn to master difficult problems. In addition, Kuhlman (1984) observed that there are similarities between "getting a joke" and "experiencing an insight about one's own patterns or psychological reactions." In this manner, humor can be very helpful. However, when used injudiciously in treatment, the use of humor with a medically ill patient can create the perception that the therapist does not understand the pain, chooses to ignore the distress the patient is experiencing, or is uncomfortable with the patient's illness, distress, or both. It is important to remember that with humor, as with any potentially important tool toward behavior change, the tool can be destructive or helpful.

7. DO: Focus treatment on complex psychological, emotional, existential, and spiritual problems.
   DON'T: Assume that treatment focuses only on superficial problems.

Laypersons rarely initially see PST as a means with which to develop answers or solutions to complex problems, such as relationship difficulties, fears of death, sexual dysfunction, or pain. Instead, they tend to associate it more with a cognitive process useful in business or making concrete decisions, such as which job to take, what dress to buy, or even which physician to choose. It is important to communicate that problem-solving skills are applicable and helpful to a wide range of complex, emotional, and interpersonal problems.

8. DO: Focus specific training and attention on solution implementation.
   DON'T: Minimally address the implementation portion of PST training.

Because so much effort is directed toward increasing the patient's positive problem orientation, expectancy for increased coping abilities, belief in the program, and rational problem-solving skills, a therapist may assume that competent thinking and positive intentions will be followed by instrumental actions. However, if there were motivation problems at other points along the way, there is a good chance that such problems will occur when the patient is faced with implementing a chosen solution. Specific attention needs to be focused on this area. In addition, actual behavioral skill deficits may be present that can preclude successful implementation of a plan, for example, if one's solution plan calls for assertive behavior, it may be important for the patient to actually practice or role play the desired action before attempting to act on his or her chosen solution. Regarding this issue, there are two important points to get across: (a) Failure is not lethal and (b) it is important to act on a decision so that performance can be evaluated.

9. DO: Adequately assess psychiatric problems that either preexisted or now coexist with the medical illness.

DON'T: Inadequately assess problems such as substance abuse or suicidal risk.

Past research has found a strong association between problem-solving deficits and suicidal ideation (Schotte & Clum, 1982, 1987). As such, PST would appear to be particularly appropriate for this potentially lethal problem. Although PST may be helpful in the long run, a careful assessment is required to examine the current potential or risk of harm for the patient, as well as the need for crisis management or emergency intervention. When substance abuse is involved, the likelihood of risk is greatly increased. As mentioned earlier in this chapter, problems with substance abuse are very likely to require adjuvant psychotherapy or pharmacological treatment in the short term. When evaluation of an individual indicates a potential for self-destructive behavior, the therapist may need to take control and actually do the problem solving for the patient until the crisis is past. In such a situation, it is likely that the patient will require frequent reevaluation throughout treatment.

10. DO: Conduct an adequate evaluation of the individual patient's assets and limitations.
    DON'T: Assume that "all patients are equal."

It is important to have a comprehensive assessment to best determine the course of a patient's treatment. For example, one patient we worked with, who had a master's degree in educational psychology, was already "intellectually" skilled in problem solving. However, she had been distorting her experience of distress as a sign that "everything" was out of her control. Continual work on her orientation skills was required throughout the training. In fact, almost every new skill-training focus became another opportunity to show the patient how her thinking was sabotaging her problem-solving efforts. It took her some time to see how challenging such thoughts was an important part of problem-solving skills. If the initial assessment was limited, a picture of a "good problem solver" would have emerged, rather than one in which her rational problem-solving skills were found to be strong, but her negative problem orientation greatly affected her overall ability to cope effectively.

11. DO: Complete all of the essential components of the protocol within the context of a flexible approach.
    DON'T: Lose sight of the protocol.

It can be very tempting to go off in many different therapeutic directions that are based on the needs of a patient. For example, it may become clear that a patient's current fear of functioning independently may be tied to fears of being abandoned. In individual therapy, it may be useful to take some time with the patient to see how these schemas developed earlier on and affected his or her life. However, this represents a diversion from PST, and if a therapist's work with the patient is confined to a very brief time-limited protocol, it may be more useful to focus on immediate ways in which the patient can continue to learn improved coping strategies, without fully understanding the development and maintenance of early maladaptive schemas. Such time restraints are often placed on the therapy situation because of the demands of research protocols, managed care guidelines, or brief hospital stays.

PST Structure

FLEXIBILITY OF THERAPY APPROACH

The PST protocol contained in this book is designed to be flexible. It can be applied in a structured and sequential method, occurring over approximately 10 sessions, as exemplified in the protocol developed for Project Genesis. Conversely, specific sessions may be selected and incorporated into a practitioner's own individual treatment plan for a given patient. In this text, topical areas that are included in the protocol are presented in the typical sequence in which they were presented in the various PST outcome studies conducted by Nezu and his colleagues. However, the length and degree of concentration devoted to any one topic may depend on the patient or the population of patients with whom it is used. The protocol may be implemented in a group, family, couples, or individual format. In the next section, we discuss particular benefits, as well as possible risks, of conducting PST with couples and groups. In chapter 11, we include a special section on how the problem-solving principles can be adopted for helping to meet the needs of cancer caregivers themselves.

The required frequency of problem-solving sessions will vary according to patients' needs, although it is advisable to include no more than 3 sessions per week, such that patients may "practice" skills in their own environment in between sessions. Table 3 serves as a quick reference guide to topics covered over the typical 10-session protocol and as a summary of the treatment components (described in the following paragraphs) that will be covered in detail in forthcoming chapters.

INTRODUCTION AND RATIONALE

We recommend that the first session be devoted to an introduction and presentation of the rationale for PST. This provides an important

TABLE 3	

Sample structure of a 10-week problem-solving therapy protocol

Session no.	Topic
1	Introduction and rationale
2	Problem orientation
3	Problem definition
4	Problem definition
5	Generation of alternatives
6	Decision making
7	Solution implementation and verification
8	Practice
9	Practice
10	Practice and termination

context and treatment philosophy for the patients. Much more than a simple definition and explanation of problem solving, this initial interaction with patients helps them to understand how thinking, feeling, and interacting in their personal relationships can help or hinder their medical treatment and consummate wellness. It is particularly important to communicate that through problem solving, patients take responsibility for their health, and not blame others for their illness. Additionally, this session provides a time to describe ground rules for treatment and expectations of both therapist and patient contributions to the collaboration of treatment.

PROBLEM ORIENTATION

The session(s) devoted to training in problem orientation contain strategies aimed at strengthening an individual's ability to accurately recognize, perceive, and better understand the problems he or she is currently confronting. Because negative emotions can hinder such skills, emotion identification and management are also important foci of this training. Moreover, training in problem orientation skills helps a patient to convert emotional arousal that was previously disabling into a useful instrument for coping.

RATIONAL PROBLEM-SOLVING SKILLS

The remaining four component skills are referred to as *rational problem-solving skills* because they are all necessary to a systematic and logical problem-solving process. This training typically follows sessions devoted to problem orientation because individuals learn to use and apply these skills more easily if they have developed some mastery in accurate problem recognition and a better understanding of how to use their emotions more effectively. They are usually taught in the suggested sequence, although individuals frequently process information by using two or more of these skills simultaneously. Additionally, there is a frequent "circling back" that occurs in order to use multiple components during the solving of a specific problem. For example, an individual may experience significant difficulty generating alternative solutions if he or she has inadequately defined a problem or has failed to identify relevant personal obstacles. Yet, the very process of attempting to generate these solutions is what may be needed to trigger the recognition that the problem was not well defined. Such a situation requires circling back to better define the problem before attempting to generate solutions.

Problem Definition and Formulation

Training in problem definition and formulation is focused on teaching patients to more accurately describe the internal and external events, situations, or individuals that are functionally contributing to their distress and to set personal goals. It is important to note that most therapists have found that the ability to define problems accurately is a complex skill, which usually requires additional therapy time. This is because teaching patients to function as personal scientists and to define problems without bias first involves strategies geared to help them accept such an approach as feasible. This may require substantial session time in and of itself. In addition, actually learning such skills requires significant practice, guidance, and reinforcement.

Generation of Alternatives

Individuals learn to generate alternatives by creatively brainstorming multiple possible ways to achieve specific goals and overcome identified obstacles. Therapeutic strategies are aimed at ways to increase the patience, creativity, and cognitive flexibility required to accomplish this skill.

Decision Making

Decision making involves learning to conduct a personal cost–benefit analysis of one's personal options. This component process individualizes the definition of the "best" solution by teaching people to recognize the consequences of their actions on their own intra- and inter-personal affairs, as well as value systems.

Solution Implementation and Verification

Solution implementation includes strategies to put thoughts and planning into actual action. Finally, solution implementation increases the accuracy and frequency with which patients self-monitor and self-reinforce their problem-solving efforts.

MAINTENANCE, GENERALIZATION, AND PRACTICE

As referred to earlier in this chapter and as indicated in Table 3, specific strategies designed to encourage practice and to increase generalization and maintenance of skills should be included in any therapy experience. Particularly with regard to PST, prevention of future episodes of anxiety and depression can significantly be minimized when individuals continue to use PST skills long after therapy termination. Thus, strategies aimed at helping individuals to "own" these skills as part of who they are and how they think are instrumental to increasing skill maintenance.

Occasionally, naive therapists have made the serious mistake of viewing PST skills training as a psychoeducational process that is not likely to instigate strong emotional attachments to a therapist or present much difficulty regarding the therapy termination process. This is not the case. Individuals who have made even a 10-week commitment at this vulnerable time in their life have placed their trust and hope in both the PST process and the therapist. As such, ending this relationship represents a loss. Strategies aimed at achieving successful conclusion to therapy focus on providing continued trust in the PST process and helping patients to trust in themselves as problem solvers.

Special Therapy Conditions: Significant Others and Groups

PST WITH SIGNIFICANT OTHERS: PARTNERS IN PROBLEM SOLVING

In chapter 2, we briefly described the initial results of Project Genesis regarding the inclusion of a significant other in the PST training protocol. Although the therapy condition that included a significant other was not shown to specifically add to the effects of treatment, there may be situations in which including significant others may be helpful. As indicated in our discussion of these findings, there may be unique aspects of this study that contribute to the lack of results. As such, it is too early to conclude that working with couples or families will not add value to the intervention. Particularly in private-practice situations, a therapist's clinical judgment may be the best current determinant of whether to include significant others in treatment. When considering applications of PST to working with couples, there are important considerations that will affect the type of strategies used and the benefits to treatment. The most minimal involvement of a significant other exists when this person is included as a "working consultant" for the purpose of evaluation, helping the patient to seek information, or giving feedback. In such a case, the significant other is a "collaborative guest of treatment." Using the analogy of a sporting event, in which the patient is the player striving to survive or win, the significant other is an *interested spectator*. When the partner or friend attends all sessions from the start of treatment in the role of a helper, as in Project Genesis, he or she acts more as a cheerleader or *coach*. In such a case he or she helps motivate, guide, and support the player. Finally, in a true couples or partners treatment, the significant other is an *equal player* with a responsibility to work hard and has a mutual personal stake in the outcome.

All three roles can and do occur in psychotherapy situations and largely depend on the context and initial reason for referral. As such, it is important to clarify the roles and responsibilities of the significant other at the very start of treatment. If the role is one of a spectator, the partner can help evaluate where the patient's problem-solving strengths and weaknesses are and provide information to the therapist and patient concerning how the patient's interactions with others may affect people close to him or her. If included in treatment as a coach, the significant other should agree to help the patient learn the problem-solving skills, reinforce the patient when he or she is actively using a skill, and suggest the use of specific skills (i.e., reminders) when the patient is experiencing distress and not utilizing the skills effectively. If included in a therapy–patient partnership, the significant other should identify situations that are problematic or troublesome for him or her and should practice the skills relevant to his or her own goals. Therapy is also likely to include mutual goals that a partnership may identify, such as "helping the children through Dad's cancer treatment."

In any of these therapeutic situations discussed, when working with significant others, it is important to provide such individuals with a personal benefit from PST. As such, caution should be exercised never to ignore the personal needs of the family members or significant others. Additionally, many medical patients come to treatment experiencing guilt and a sense of burden to their families. They may have a heightened sensitivity to hearing criticism and view their own coping difficulties as additional burdens. Significant others, caregivers, and other family members may also feel particularly guilty or hesitant to talk about their feelings. Caregivers or individuals engaged as coaches may feel additionally burdened by the homework and requirements of training. It is important to communicate to significant others in all of the roles discussed that their participation in PST can help improve their own quality of life as well. At times, the problems worked on in treatment may well focus on improving family relationships and communication patterns.

PST WITH GROUPS

Terms such as group therapy, group counseling, or group skills training can all carry different connotations, and, depending on the theoretical underpinnings of the group, use different therapy goals. To conduct PST optimally in a group format, aspects of group therapy, group counseling, and group skills training should all be included. Because there is a specific group agenda to increase problem-solving skills, there is clearly a group *skills training* component that will be focused on while learning and practicing new skills, as well as actively confronting problems. *Group counseling* characteristics of focusing on immediate environmental problems and short-term issues can provide an efficient short-term approach to problem solving. Such an approach can be used when therapeutic needs require constructing a PST training group for anything from a 1-day workshop intervention to a 10-week brief psychotherapy protocol. If focused more on immediate environmental problems with a similar theme for all group members, it may be possible to have groups led by trained facilitators who are not necessarily licensed psychologists. PST *group therapy* allows a group to focus on more long-term interpersonal and characterological problems in the relatively "safe atmosphere" of a small therapeutic community. Such therapy situations require the leadership of an experienced clinician who can assess individuals in the group who may either facilitate or block the treatment of others and who is knowledgeable in strategies to manage such individuals.

D'Zurilla and Nezu (in press) described the advantages of a group program to include motivating effects of group discussion, sharing of ideas and experiences, modeling, social support, social reinforcement, and more efficient use of therapy instructors or facilitators. Throughout the remainder of the book, at the end of each chapter, we include clinical tips regarding the application of certain problem-solving strategies for groups. However, one important overall strategy is to use the group setting to increase support and reinforcement for learning PST. A group format can provide a useful analogue to everyday life in which new ways of coping can be encouraged and former destructive interpersonal habits can be discouraged.

A major reason to implement PST in a group setting is practical in nature—many hospital or community-based programs may already have formed groups that meet on a regular basis. In such cases, PST may be a meaningful approach to use. However, certain individuals may seek a more private context in which to discuss personal issues. Therefore, a therapist needs to be flexible in the manner in which PST is conducted.

Summary

In this chapter, we provided an overview of PST for cancer patients by discussing various general clinical issues, including the structure of PST, the assessment guidelines, the therapist–patient relationship, and the use of adjunctive therapeutic strategies. PST goals were described as helping distressed cancer patients to (a) identify previous and current life situations that serve to increase the intensity and frequency of their distress, (b) reduce the extent to which distressful emotions negatively affect their current and future attempts at coping, (c) increase the effectiveness of their problem-solving coping attempts concerning current problem situations, and (d) teach skills that will enable them to deal more effectively with future problems. We characterized PST as appropriate for all cancer patients who are experiencing emotional distress or who have difficulties making treatment decisions. On the basis of the wide range of difficulties that cancer and its treatment engender, PST may be a particularly useful means of learning to cope with these diverse problems.

A positive therapist–patient relationship was posited to be an important component of this and any other psychosocial intervention. Various characteristics of the therapist were outlined that may potentially mediate the effectiveness of the treatment with any given patient.

PST was characterized as comprising three major stages: assessment, intervention, and generalization training. If feasible, assessment should entail a comprehensive interview and the completion of various self-report measures cutting across issues of emotional distress symptomatology, quality of life, and problem-solving coping ability.

We offered a variety of suggested inventories geared to address these areas.

PST intervention primarily encompasses training in the five major problem-solving processes: problem orientation, problem definition and formulation, generation of alternatives, decision making, and solution implementation and verification. Chapters 4–9 were written with the intention of providing a detailed treatment manual to aid the therapist in conducting this approach. In addition, however, we advocate using a variety of therapeutic strategies that can facilitate skill acquisition. These include didactic instruction, handouts, teaching metaphors, prompting, shaping, modeling, behavioral rehearsal, homework assignments, reinforcement, and feedback.

We also provided a list of problem-solving therapy "Do's and Don'ts" that underscore important therapeutic features when conducting this approach and applying this approach to special therapy conditions.

Critical Elements of Training

4

Therapeutic Goals of the Introductory Session

The goals of an introductory session and initial presentation of problem-solving therapy (PST) to the patient include the following: (a) to establish a positive relationship (i.e., communicate warmth, trust, caring, and respect), or for patients already engaged in treatment, to present the training as redirecting the treatment focus to develop certain coping skills for decreasing cancer-related distress; (b) to present an overview and rationale of the program (e.g., why the focus will be on problem solving, what the patient will get out of it, how PST will uniquely be adapted to a given patient's experience, and what will actually occur during the training); (c) to encourage optimism (i.e., have the patient leave the session with the expectation that this training will be of help); and (d) to communicate that the therapist see the person's potential for effective coping (e.g., framing observed deficits within the context of a balanced approach that also identifies strengths and areas in which practice might be needed). For group treatments, the therapist's communication can take the form of statements regarding how the different strengths and weaknesses of each patient can work to benefit each other.

Establishing a Positive Relationship

We have found it clinically useful to use the following format in establishing a rapport with new patients who have been referred for PST. The therapist should begin by introducing him- or herself (e.g., one's professional background and current role regarding this patient's overall treatment) and then presenting a brief overview of anticipated activities (e.g., "You and I will be working together to try to reduce some of the distress that you are currently experiencing").

Early in the initial session, it is important to ask a patient about his or her cancer diagnosis (e.g., what type and when the diagnosis was made). More important, questions should focus on the person's own cancer experience (e.g. "Tell me about you" vs. "Give me the specifics of your medical treatment"). This approach has been reported by patients as comforting because of the relief that someone in their life is not reluctant to discuss the impact of cancer when so many friends and family members are avoidant and fearful of the topic. It is important when discussing a patient's cancer experience to include questions concerning how his or her life has changed (e.g., what is his or her predominant reaction, the reaction of the family, and the effects on his or her job and friends). When sessions are attended by a significant other, or reported problems involve a significant other, it may be important to ask about the impact cancer has had on the relationship with the other individuals in the patient's life.

During a patient's responses to such questions, it is important to use those counseling methods geared to enhance the therapist–patient relationship (e.g., reflection of content and feeling: "It sounds like you felt your whole world fell apart"). Finally, as in almost all treatment approaches, it is critical to any therapeutic relationship to display warmth, support, genuine interest, and a sense of commitment to the patient.

People are understandably cautious about seeing a mental health professional when they have a physical, rather than a mental, illness. As such, it is important to emphasize one's role as a teacher (i.e., to teach the patient how to sort through this experience and to learn new skills) as compared with "psychoanalyzing" him or her. In addition, it is important to underscore the notion of teamwork and mutual respect (e.g., "You will help me to understand how your life has changed and the new problems you have encountered, and I will show you how people can learn to become more effective at solving many of these types of problems").

Presenting the Rationale

The introduction of a patient to PST will require that the therapist discuss the importance of psychological interventions in treating cancer as a chronic illness. As such, when therapists present an initial introduction and rationale for PST, it is important to first consider how best to incorporate these strategies into a patient's overall treatment plan. Then, an overview of the program can be provided and attempts made to facilitate patient motivation. We believe that the session in which the rationale of PST is introduced is particularly important, in that the success of any therapeutic endeavor is based in part on the degree to which a patient understands and accepts the underlying precepts and philosophy of a given intervention approach. Thus, it is important for the therapist during this aspect of training to present a comprehensive picture, in "layterms," of the rationale behind PST. However, attempts should be made to prevent any didactic component being viewed as a lecture. Rather, this information needs to be conveyed within a therapeutic context and with many examples drawn from the real world.

"Why Should I Learn Problem Solving When I'm Diagnosed With Cancer?"

This is a question that we are often asked by a cancer patient during an initial referral visit. To help the reader, throughout this chapter, as well as in the remaining chapters making up the book, we provide examples of how a therapist may actually state his or her rationale to the patient, in other words, how to answer this question. However, we urge readers to remember the importance of adapting wording and language to be in concert with each individual patient's developmental, educational, and cultural background. Recognizing this need for individualized adaptation, we recommend the following major areas of explanation for inclusion into the therapist's explanation of PST.

CANCER AS A MAJOR LIFE STRESSOR

When conceptualizing cancer as a major life stressor, the therapist may wish to describe how major life events (e.g., medical illness, natural disasters, unemployment, and divorce) often create additional problems. For example, experiencing a divorce might represent a living relocation. This might also include new environs for children, which means making new decisions about schools, having to find new places to shop and bank, and engaging in new social activities. Emotions are often mixed and involve many different people. Problems with finances and extended family members are also common. When experiencing a life event such as cancer and its treatment, as with most major life stressors, individuals will encounter both major and minor problems. These problems can cumulatively lead to distress. As such, cancer can be seen as directly leading to distress. Distress leads to more problems, such as how to reduce the negative feelings or troublesome thoughts—this additional burden can create a downward spiral of cognitive and emotional reactions, such as despair and hopelessness. As an ancient Persian proverb suggests, "If fortune turns against you, even jelly breaks your teeth."

Significant distress, such as that described earlier, can at times even lead to less than optimal cancer treatment (e.g., missed appointments or poor compliance with diet recommendations). When discussing the deleterious consequences of patient distress, it is often helpful to use specific and relevant examples from each patient's actual report of difficulties. For example, an individual may be coming to treatment concerned about new problems at work that are a result of the cancer treatment. Such examples, if incorporated, will provide relevance and meaning for the patient regarding how problem-solving coping is tied into his or her own unique difficulties. Finally, stress also appears to have a negative effect on one's immune system. Thus, poor coping may lead to poor health outcomes. When discussing the association between psychological and emotional coping and actual health outcomes, it should be underscored that taking responsibility for one's health and well-being does not mean accepting blame for the illness. Rather, effective stress management skills provide one with the best chance for well-being in light of all of the other biomedical and environmental variables that influence health and disease.

MODERATORS OF STRESS

Moderators of stress are factors that help reduce, minimize, or prevent distress. The discussion and explanation of stress moderators should begin with a brief description of social support and resources (e.g., lots of money reduces financial worries regarding health costs and supportive family and friends help to reduce emotional distress), the differing types of effective coping strategies (e.g., prayer, humor, exercise, or a positive spirit such as a "fighting back attitude"), and the role of problem-solving coping. The introduction of problem-solving coping skills at this point in the rationale should underscore the notion that solving even a few cancer-related problems can break a chain of cumulative stress and can enhance one's overall quality of life.

DESCRIPTION OF PROBLEM SOLVING

The most parsimonious definition of this construct is that problem solving is a set of skills or tools that people can use to resolve problems and difficulties encountered in daily living. In addition, we typically explain to patients that many people possess some of these skills, but need practice with others, particularly when they are experiencing a new stressor. Finally, even for people who have excellent problem-solving skills developed at work or as a function of their education, they often do not apply these skills to situations involving personal problems or when strong emotions are involved. Yet, ironically, these are times when such skills can be most useful and effective.

When a significant other is involved as a coach or partner, the therapist can emphasize how problem-solving skills are useful for daily living in general and, therefore, are useful to anyone who is learning the skills. We have found that people accept the concept that oncology professionals (i.e., physicians and nurses) serve as "medical problem solvers" and that people with cancer can function as "personal problem solvers."

THE PROVEN EFFECTIVENESS OF PST

Explaining to the patient that substantial research has shown this approach to be effective can increase his or her confidence in treatment. Furthermore, knowledge that this training has helped other people to reduce their depression, anxiety, and distress associated with medical or rehabilitative problems can increase patient motivation (see chapter 2 for review of supporting research of PST).

Problem-solving skills are similar to other types of skills such as learning how to drive, how to play a musical instrument, or how to play sports. It is important that the therapist explains to the patient that to learn to solve problems effectively, PST (a) requires some instruction, (b) involves practice, and (c) may feel awkward in the beginning, which is similar to all new skills.

At this point, one of the roles of a significant other, as described in the previous chapter, can be emphasized. For example, it can be noted that people benefit from an observer's feedback, a coach's encouragement, or a fellow player's collaboration for most sports, musical instrument skills, or physical rehabilitation. It is important to emphasize that the participation of such individuals can significantly enhance the quality of life for both persons.

Below is an example of an introduction to problem solving that combines these points into an introduction:

> People may have difficulty coping with an illness like cancer because it is a major problem that they never had to cope with before. A large range of emotional reactions like fear, anger, and sadness are normal and expected . . . emotional reactions or negative feelings always occur with problems. This can lead to more problems, because major changes in our life are like that— they can, and do, affect everything that we do in our day-to-day life. When feelings of being overwhelmed lead to not wanting to even think about problems, this can lead to avoidance. Avoidance of problems almost always makes them worse. People who are good problem solvers generally don't avoid problems, but they try to stay calm and work on finding solutions to some of these problems, even if all of them can't be solved.
>
> Often the stress associated with cancer leads to "emotional problem solving"; that is, decisions that are based on strong emotions, not rational thinking. Making decisions in this way, often on the spur of the moment, rarely leads to the best results for you—you have enough problems, you don't need any more right now. Cancer also means that you will have to make many important decisions. Decisions that are important for you and that need to be based on rational thinking. Thus, training in problem solving can lead to improved quality of life, now and after cancer treatment.

After providing a rationale for PST, the therapist can inform the patient that training involves understanding, learning, and practicing five component skill areas (i.e., problem orientation, problem definition and formulation, generation of alternatives, decision making, and solution implementation and verification). A brief overview of these problem-solving operations can then be provided, the therapist making certain to include concrete and appropriate examples when possible. The following is an example of how the problem-solving component processes can be described in laypersons' terms:

> You and I will work together to give you the most effective ways to manage all the stresses of illness. We will start by looking at how you react to problems and understand your own emotions (a relevant example, such as "fighting spirit" or "optimism" can be offered here as a concrete example of problem orientation). Training in this area, called *problem orientation,* focuses on how you react to and think about problems. In general, this problem-solving approach will help you to learn to do the following: how to look at problems (e.g., as a challenge vs. a threat), how to perceive problems in an adaptive manner (e.g., a "head-on" approach vs. avoidance), how to improve your problem-solving style (e.g., thoughtful and systematic vs. impulsive), how to define problems and set goals, how to understand why the

situation is a problem, how to identify accurately major obstacles, how to set realistic goals, how to invent and to create new solutions to problems, how to use brainstorming techniques, how to make good decisions, how to conduct a cost–benefit analysis of consequences, how to focus on short- and long-term consequences, how to monitor and evaluate the outcome of a solution, how to carry out a solution plan, how to monitor the consequences (e.g., balancing a checkbook when keeping to a strict budget and weighing oneself when on a diet), and how to evaluate the outcome.

Moreover, we view these skills as a general way of approaching and solving life's problems. In essence, you will learn a set of skills that can be applied to all types of problems—those that you are experiencing now and those in the future. To a large extent, it's like the old saying, "Give a person a fish, he eats for a day . . . teach a person to fish, he eats for a lifetime." In other words, PST is like learning to fish—you will be able to use these skills throughout your lifetime.

It is important to emphasize that problem solving (a) is a systematic and orderly approach to coping with stress and (b) helps to facilitate flexibility and creativity. Next, the goals of PST can be discussed and provided as a handout (see Figure 4.1). These goals include the following: (a) training persons with cancer to be effective problem solvers; (b) decreasing emotional and psychological distress; (c) facilitating a patient's overall quality of life and adjustment; and (d) increasing a patient's sense of control. If a significant other or family member is present, the therapist can outline specific goals for such individuals. These may include the following: (a) helping significant others to manage their role as support persons or caregivers; (b) managing the changes and stressors that have occurred for them; and (c) using the problem-solving model to help better deal with commonly occurring feelings experienced by significant others such as fear, worry, anger, and guilt.

ENCOURAGE OPTIMISM AND A SENSE OF CONTROL

It is important to facilitate a patient's sense of optimism and belief that one can regain control of one's life. The therapist should try to identify and point out examples of potentially effective problem-solving attempts with the information that the patient provides. In addition, the therapist should acknowledge that cancer affects the "whole person," not just the body. It should be emphasized that people's overall response to problems can work either for or against them; the goal of PST is to increase the chance that a patient's reactions will work for him or her.

FIGURE 4.1

GOALS OF PROBLEM SOLVING

❏   *To improve problem solving*

❏   *To decrease distress*

❏   *To improve quality of life*

❏   *To increase sense of control*

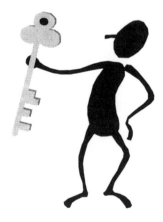

Goals of problem solving handout.

The following is a sample explanation of the earlier points:

We know that people who are facing cancer are physically facing a disease. But just as important is the notion that people facing cancer are also *psychologically* facing a disease of fear. Some doctors work to cure the cancer and heal your body. We work to minimize the fears and help you to improve your thoughts and spirits. With diseases like cancer, the body hurts, but the whole person suffers. We want to help the person to suffer much less— not just the body, but the whole person! We have helped many people like yourself to get more out of life and cope with very difficult situations in their lives through learning to become effective problem solvers. Having cancer affects everything. In addition to medically treating the cancer, we think it is also important to treat you as a whole person—your mind and your spirit!

COMMUNICATE PERSON'S POTENTIAL FOR COMPETENCE

It is particularly important to reinforce a patient's current competencies in various areas of living to enhance motivation for optimally engaging in PST. Furthermore, it is important to make analogies to the person's obvious abilities (e.g., job, housekeeping, or volunteer work). If a patient appears very pessimistic, the therapist should emphasize the importance of using such emotions as a signal for the need to use problem solving (i.e., a problem exists).

GROUND RULES AND THERAPY EXPECTATIONS

Many patients may not be familiar with a skill development approach to psychotherapy and subsequently be unaware of therapy expectations. As such, it is important to discuss with patients several "ground rules" of the approach, along with other "standard" therapy issues such as confidentiality and informed consent. We have found it useful to include such a discussion of session timing and frequency, as well as expectations of homework between sessions as part of PST ground rules. It can be additionally useful to obtain mutual agreement with patients concerning joint responsibilities. These include the following.

Therapist Responsibilities

The therapist should agree to draw on all training, knowledge of scientific literature, and clinical experience to best help the cancer patient.

Patient Responsibilities

The patient needs to agree to "give it his or her best shot," do the homework, practice skills, keep appointments, and let the therapist know of problems or disappointments with treatment. These same rules would also apply to patients in a group.

Case Examples for This Book

To illustrate the various techniques used throughout the text with patient examples, we continuously discuss the cases of Gary and Terry. These two patients will provide an ongoing clinical context for the various illustrations. In keeping with the theme of this chapter (i.e., the first session), we introduce Gary and Terry in the following paragraphs.

TERRY

Terry is a 34-year-old divorced woman of average build who appears her age. Because of her mother's diagnosis of breast cancer 14 years ago, Terry had routinely conducted monthly self-breast exams. Eight months prior to seeking psychotherapy, Terry discovered a lump in her right breast. She was diagnosed with breast cancer after several tests and two medical opinions. Within 1 month of diagnosis, she had a radical mastectomy. Although her cancer was in an early stage in which it appeared to be contained in a solid tumor, Terry decided against breast-conserving surgery. She attributed this decision to her fear of recurrence and to the lack of certainty that a lumpectomy would "get it all." Subsequently, she did not comply with her physician's advice to have adjuvant chemotherapy. Terry reasoned that she had her entire breast removed, and, therefore, all of the cancer was likely to be gone. Terry wanted to put the cancer behind her and "go on with her life."

In the initial evaluation by the psychologist, Terry described her current difficulties as focused on "how to put the pieces back together and put the cancer behind her." Since her diagnosis and treatment, several other areas of her life seem to have been affected by her experience with cancer.

Physically, Terry looked healthy. She had not yet decided whether to have reconstructive surgery, but she currently had a prosthesis that was undetectable by others. This was particularly troubling to her because people regarded her as having fully recovered from her diagnosis. Hence, she did not feel that she had adequate social support from friends or coworkers who have forgotten what she is "going through." She frequently became angry and irritated with them, although she did not communicate these feelings. When she was at home, she was faced with the scars and the loss of her breast. She did not allow herself to look at her naked body in the mirror, and she did not undress with the light on. Showering was problematic because she had to cleanse the scars and the surrounding area. She cried frequently when she was at home alone.

Terry had described herself as an independent, self-sufficient, career-oriented woman prior to her diagnosis. As a result of the financial burden of medical treatment and the loss of income from several months of work, Terry was forced to move out of her apartment and return to her parents' home. In addition to losing her financial independence and relinquishing her sense of control to the medical staff, she also lost her privacy and had to reacclimate herself to her parents' constant company. Living at her parents' home infringed on her social life as her parents expected her to spend time with the family and to inform them of her whereabouts. Terry had difficulty describing her feelings with regard to moving into her parents' home. She expressed guilt and embarrassment for being "selfish" and "suffocated," rather than being entirely grateful and receptive to her parents' attempts to make her comfortable. She did acknowledge that she was thankful for her parents' support and accommodations, but she wished that she was able to function independently. Although Terry and her mother had always been close, moving into her parents' home changed the relationship "back to being her little girl rather than her friend." Overall, she did not feel that she had adequate social support from friends, coworkers, or family to help her with her emotional rehabilitation.

In addition to her concerns about her body image, her financial difficulties, and her lack of independence, Terry had worries about her future. She had been divorced for 2 years after 12 years of an "emotionally numb" marriage. Her ex-husband, Jack, was a high-school sweetheart whom she dated for 4 years before they married. By the time she and Jack divorced, they had little in common. He had completed 2 years of college but was not interested in pursuing a career. They enjoyed different activities and led essentially separate lives. Terry finally left him when he admitted to having an affair. Although she was not particularly surprised, nor upset about the end of their relationship, she did fear spending the rest of her life alone. Her diagnosis of cancer, decreased self-esteem, and poor self-image, compounded with her previously existing fear of remaining single, were additional causes for distress. She found herself feeling less comfortable interacting with men and was unsure of how to address her "deformity" with them. At the time of the intake interview, she stated that she had little to no desire for sexual intimacy.

Terry withdrew from social activities that she had previously enjoyed, such as going to clubs, going golfing with coworkers in her office, or attending her book club. She found that she was less interested in these activities and lacked enthusiasm for her career as well. As a real estate agent, she was constantly having to interact with other people and was spending a lot of time traveling in her car. Prior to her diagnosis, Terry considered herself to be a social person who enjoyed the company of others. Presently, she preferred to be alone. She postponed working for the maximum time that her disability insurance allowed her but then had to return because of her financial situation.

Terry presented with increasing anxiety during the course of the interview as manifested by fidgeting, increasingly rapid speech, and a tense expression on her face. She was also tearful and desperate at times, which was appropriate to the topic. Terry did not endorse any suicidal ideation or use of controlled or illegal substances. Her coping techniques included talking to her high-school friend who lived 10 hours away, listening to music, and writing in her journal. Overall, she agreed that her coping ability was not adequate to overcome the distress she had been experiencing since her diagnosis of breast cancer.

GARY

Gary is a 62-year-old married man of moderate-to-slightly-overweight build who appears older than his age. During an annual physical examination required by his job, Gary's physician detected that his spleen was enlarged. After several investigational studies, Gary was diagnosed with chronic myelogenous leukemia and the Philadelphia chromosome abnormality. Carriers of this chromosome abnormality require more aggressive treatment than those with chronic myelogenous leukemia who do not have this abnormality. High-dose chemotherapy is indicated promptly, prior to the disease reaching the blastic or acute phase. Contact with Gary was initiated by the psychologist 1 month postdiagnosis in response to a consultation to determine his eligibility for a bone marrow transplant.

Gary had an extensive medical history including high blood pressure, myocardial infarction at the age of 51, panic attacks, and excessive alcohol use. He described himself as a "nervous person" and admitted to not handling stress well. His panic attacks had been managed by taking anxiolytic medication as needed, with the last episode occurring 3 years ago. For the past 8 years, Gary continued to attend Alcoholics Anonymous (AA) meetings and had maintained contact with his sponsor. The last lapse in sobriety occurred 6 years ago. However, Gary began to doubt his ability to cope adequately with his recent diagnosis of cancer and to remain sober.

Although he has been married for 24 years, Gary describes his relationship as being historically "unstable." After 5 years of marriage, Gary's wife, Celia, had an affair, which led to their first separation of 3 months. They had temporarily separated again for 6 months, prior to Gary's enrollment in AA. This separation was attributed to his periodic violent outbursts that occurred while he was heavily intoxicated. Gary and his wife did not have children of their own, though Celia had two children from a previous relationship. Gary did not establish a close relationship with either of these children. He considered his wife to be supportive of concrete needs, such as transportation and physical presence, but not of emotional needs. Gary stated that they have not been sexually active since his diagnosis because of his wife's fear of causing him harm through intimate contact. Gary believes that this "fear" is an excuse for "pushing him away."

In the rural area where Gary lives, he is responsible for supervising workers in a chemical plant. Gary believes that the development of his leukemia was a result of exposure to chemicals for many years. He expressed some anger toward his coworkers' and boss's lack of compassion for his diagnosis. Several men with whom Gary worked with over the years had faced a diagnosis of cancer. Gary believes that he deserved some attention from his coworkers and boss after his many years of service to this company.

With the rising cost of health care, Gary and Celia are facing financial difficulties. His medical insurance is unwilling to cover the cost of a bone marrow transplant at his hospital of choice, if the treatment is indicated. Therefore, his wife would have to incur the costs of hotel fees and travel expenses if she is to accompany him. Furthermore, she would be unable to continue to work for the minimum of 5 weeks of his treatment. Once Gary is able to return home, he would be unable to work for approximately 6 months. He will not be able to return to his job, regardless of the treatment he receives. However, he was guaranteed a desk job if he becomes well enough to resume work.

The purpose of the initial interview with Gary was to establish the likelihood of his compliance with the rigid medical regimen necessary for a successful transplant. The standard physical examination suggested that Gary's organs were functioning well enough to sustain the stress of a transplant. However, the physicians were concerned about the possibility of Gary resuming alcohol consumption, which would jeopardize his liver functioning. Obviously, engaging in reckless and self-destructive behavior would compromise the likelihood of a successful recovery posttransplant.

Gary acknowledged his fear of returning to alcohol as a coping mechanism. He stated that he felt that his cancer diagnosis was a punishment for his past behavior, and he did not want to repeat his mistakes. Therefore, he was open and receptive to learning new ways of coping with his diagnosis, its treatment, and the many additional stresses he was facing.

Although Gary's affect was blunted, he indicated that he felt very sad, guilty, and angry about his plight. When learning of his diagnosis, Gary immediately considered committing suicide by ingesting pills; however, he had no history of attempts. Furthermore, no active suicidal ideation was present. Yet, Gary reserved that if he experienced excessive, uncontrollable pain, coupled with no treatment alternatives, he would again consider taking his own life by overdosing on pain medication. He often experienced feelings of worthlessness with regard to his marital relationship and his inability to generate income. Because of his medical illness, combined with depressive symptomatology, Gary experiences fatigue throughout the day. In addition, he endorses physical and cognitive manifestations of anxiety that prevent him from gaining restful nights of sleep.

Gary claims that he is not overly concerned with a reoccurrence of panic attacks because they have been controlled by the medication. Furthermore, he has learned some methods of relaxation, which include distraction, imagery, and taking hot baths. Wood carving is his favorite hobby that he engages in frequently in his free time. These techniques, in combination with his medication, have been moderately helpful during stressful situations up until his diagnosis. Gary is unable to continue wood carving because of the heightened risk of infection during chemotherapy, which, unfortunately, limits his options for distraction.

Since his diagnosis, Gary describes himself as being impulsive and reacting to situations immediately, often with undesirable consequences. When his affect reflects his emotions, it tends to be in situations in which he is feeling frustrated or angry. He expressed frustration when describing his physical limitations and restrictions and feeling "out of control of everything" that was important to him.

Many of Gary's emotional reactions to his cancer diagnosis were not uncommon. Given his limited range of coping techniques and his limited range of social support, he was assessed to be at an increased risk for relapsing into alcohol use. However, Gary indicated a will to live and to pursue aggressive medical treatment and not to "repeat my mistakes." He expressed willingness to commit to ongoing PST to increase his coping skills and to help him gain a sense of control. The recommendation given to the oncology team was that if Gary engaged and participated in PST, the likelihood of his compliance with the medical regimen would greatly increase.

Summary

In this chapter, we provided recommendations for the first therapy session—presentation of the purpose, rationale, structure, and content of PST. In addition to a description and an overview of the problem-solving process, this session underscores the use of relevant personal examples from patients' lives to help them better understand how stress and coping are related to the cancer experience. Additionally, patients are provided with an increased awareness of how improved coping skills can contribute to successful survival.

We also described the importance of focusing on increasing a patient's sense of control and optimism to maximize motivation. Ground rules for PST therapy, in addition to common psychotherapy guidelines, were discussed. Again, we cannot emphasize strongly enough the need to make this session as positive as possible for the patient. Answering all questions competently, providing understandable rationales, using meaningful and relevant examples, and enhancing the patient's motivation are important activities of the problem-solving therapist during this introductory session. If a patient appears hesitant to continue, more time needs to be devoted to explaining this approach and to making it applicable and relevant to his or her life.

Beginning with this chapter, we end each training chapter with the following "boxes" to enhance familiarity with implementing PST: key training points, suggested handouts, homework assignments, and group tips. As mentioned earlier, the list of group tips provides hints on how to adapt various training exercises for groups, as well as to highlight those strategies especially conducive to group participation.

Key Training Points

- Establish a positive relationship
- Present PST rationale
- Ask about reasons for seeking psychological assistance regarding a medical diagnosis
- Explain problem-solving model of stress, "cancer as a major life stressor"
- Describe how stressors can be managed through problem solving
- Describe content and efficacy of PST
- Compare PST training to learning other skills
- Encourage optimism
- Communicate patient potential for competence
- Explain ground rules and therapy expectations

Suggested Handouts

- A notebook (e.g., three-ring looseleaf-type binder for patients to store weekly handouts and homework sheets) that should be brought to each session.
- Project goals (Figure 4.1)
- Record of Coping Attempts worksheets (Figure 3.1 from chapter 3)

Homework

- As indicated in the previous chapter, we recommend that homework assignments be provided for every session while the patient is engaged in PST. If the therapist believes that a homework assignment is too advanced or that a patient is incapable of carrying out the homework that we have suggested for a specific session, it is important to give even a small assignment that will need to be addressed and completed between sessions. Our suggestion for the introductory session is to have the patient complete at least two Record of Coping Attempts worksheets (Figure 3.1) and bring them into the next session. This will provide important information concerning how he or she currently reacts to problems.
- The problem-solving therapist should plan to review the homework and have it available for reference as training begins in problem orientation. To maximize the likelihood that the patient will complete the homework, it is important to review the homework sheets that will be used and to have the patient practice filling one out with the therapist's help. Regarding the coping attempts homework form, it is important to review it in detail and to provide examples for the patient to help him or her differentiate thoughts from feelings.

Group Tips

- Allow time to establish a positive relationship between group members through personal introductions and discussion of personal expectations of the group.
- Engage group members in providing examples of how major stressors can lead to an increase in minor stressors and additional problems applicable to them.
- Engage group members in providing examples of moderators of stress.
- As a strategy to communicate personal competencies, ask group members to state one ability of which they are proud. This will provide the therapist and other group members with

a relevant example area with which to draw on for later references to recognizing competency.

■ Carefully observe the group for individuals who may serve to draw the group offtrack, attack other group members, or demand excessive attention. Make modifications in ground rules to compensate for such difficulties. Present such rules to the group in a matter-of-fact manner that communicates the common use of such rules.

III | PROBLEM-SOLVING COPING SKILLS TRAINING

Problem Orientation 5

The presence of a positive and constructive cognitive framework when approaching problems is crucial to successful problem solving (A. M. Nezu & Perri, 1989). Helping patients to adopt such a realistic optimism, however, can be an especially challenging task for clinicians who work with individuals who are overwhelmed with the emotional experience of cancer. Such patients may simultaneously experience emotions of fear, anger, sadness, guilt, and embarrassment. These emotions may operatively interfere with one's information processing and tend to overshadow objective and constructive thinking. Following a diagnosis of cancer, it is not unusual to observe such emotional interference even in individuals who have typically used more rational thinking in past stressful situations. In other words, cancer may have a unique and profound effect on one's ability to cope successfully. In an attempt to process the information surrounding cancer and its treatment, as well as these profound interruptions in coping ability, some people may attribute their distress to internal factors such as weakness or faulty traits. Conversely, other individuals may perceive cancer to be an extreme situational problem for which psychological improvement is not possible. As such, they may view a complete cancer cure as the only means by which to alleviate distress.

Development of a more positive orientation to problems involves a combination of cognitive and emotional factors. These factors include the following: (a) acceptance of problems and stressful experiences as predictable and "normal" reactions to stressors such as cancer, (b) recognition that cancer is a complex phenomenon and that cancer treatment involves significant patient participation in treatment, (c) adoption of emotional regulation skills (e.g., affect recognition and use of emotions as personal tools in the problem-solving process), and (d) expectation of successful survival. This latter issue may involve the goal of "psychological survival," especially when physical survival or disease cure is not possible.

During the initial patient assessment and treatment period, care should be taken to pay close attention to the patient's reactions to explanations and training in problem orientation. Through such careful observation, the therapist is able to evaluate areas of weakness, as well as to identify where there is a need to spend more time on a specific aspect of training. It is important to recognize that, when moving on to training in the other problem-solving skills, an individual's cognitive and emotional reaction styles can be habituated and well learned. Changing such precepts, views, and beliefs often requires repeated practice. As such, it is helpful to pinpoint areas of vulnerability that the therapist may view as an impediment to adopting a positive orientation for a given patient. Then, frequent reference can be made as negative attitudes, cognitive distortions, and self-defeating interpersonal patterns reemerge throughout training. Furthermore, new ways of thinking, or exhibiting an increase in a positive orientation, can deliberately be reinforced. Although the content in problem orientation training typically requires only several sessions to cover adequately all of the information and assessment necessary to continue with the protocol, it is important to address a patient's tendency to relapse into former ways of thinking or viewing problems throughout the treatment process.

Overview

The goals of training in problem orientation include the following: (a) to facilitate a positive and constructive problem-solving orientation that is focused on survival; (b) to emphasize the idea that problem solving is a viable means of coping with problems; (c) to reduce cognitive distortions or faulty belief patterns that might interfere with effective problem solving; and (d) to facilitate acceptance of emotional reactions and to "use" emotions as an important problem-solving tool.

Presenting the Rationale

When introducing problem orientation, it is helpful for the therapist to reinforce the importance of understanding the way in which people focus attention, predict, think about, and interpret the problems that they experience. Furthermore, how one thinks about his or her own abilities to manage emerging problems effectively should also be underscored. When current examples that are relevant to an individual's day-to-day life are used to emphasize these points, the therapist accomplishes two major objectives: (a) The patient's cognitive and emotional experience is "validated," and (b) the therapist provides a reason for why problem orientation is important for this specific patient.

PROBLEM ORIENTATION: CASE EXAMPLE

Clinical Case: Gary

Focusing on one of the case examples previously described in chapter 4, we use Gary's experience as an opportunity to indicate how problem orientation can be introduced to a patient. Gary and his therapist identified his past use of alcohol as a means of numbing negative emotions and of avoiding the interpersonal problems that he experienced. Although his sobriety in recent years had provided him with an increased ability to tolerate most day-to-day hassles, his recent cancer encounter had resulted in his experiencing profound feelings of anger and guilt. He viewed his illness as evidence that he had "no control over anything in his life" and viewed himself as a failure in his role of husband and family provider. Gary experienced a strong pull to avoid these feelings and to numb the painful emotional experiences he was enduring. He began to assign negative interpretations to the behavior of his wife, stepchildren, and coworkers. For example, Gary's past outbursts of anger and current dysphoria were often followed by other people distancing themselves from him. Gary viewed this reaction as evidence that he was unsupported. These distortions were identified during the initial problem orientation sessions. However, the tendency to associate painful feelings with evidence of being out of control and being rejected by others was a continual theme that emerged throughout Gary's treatment. The dialogue that follows provides an example of how the various strategies and techniques associated with problem orientation were explained to Gary as he described some of the current problems that served as an impetus for his therapy referral. In Gary's case, these distortions and underlying beliefs were well learned and reinforced over time by the way in which he perceived, understood, and ultimately interacted with others. Therefore, even when focusing on other skills, it was important for Gary's therapist to continually review the highlights of training in problem orientation and to frequently use homework assignments for facilitating learning. In the following dialogue, while introducing problem orientation, the therapist had asked Gary about some of the particularly troubling problems that he has recently experienced. In this dialogue, Gary begins by talking about the level of help and support that he perceives he is getting from his wife, Celia.

GARY.   She's been good—you know, taking me to chemo appointments and for tests and so on, but she doesn't understand. I have emotional needs and she just doesn't get it!

THERAPIST.   You sound angry.

GARY.   I am! I feel like screaming or something. I know she goes out of her way to help with the appointments, and taking care of things at home, and insurance, and making sure about my diet and all that; but she can't handle my feelings, and she pulls away from me—I feel like screaming at her to just stop and take care of me—she uses all the stuff that she's doing like an excuse to stay away from me.

THERAPIST.   And you would like to see this situation changed?

GARY.   Well, I'm grateful she does this stuff, but I still feel like I'm all alone with this.

THERAPIST.   The way you describe things, it seems that Celia is taking care of all the "business" of cancer, and you're carrying all the feelings about it. Have you talked to her about this?

GARY.   What good would that do? She'd probably get mad and say that she's doing so much and that I should know how much she cares—but sometimes I think that she stays so busy so she doesn't have to feel guilty staying away from me. All this talk she does about caring for me—I wonder how much she'd care if I didn't have a big insurance policy.

THERAPIST.   So you have yourself convinced at this point that Celia's motives are based solely on greed—do you really believe that?

GARY.   No . . . I don't know . . . I just feel so out of control sometimes—I wish I could just think straight.

THERAPIST.   Let's slow down a bit here. When you say "I wish I could think straight," I think you mean "If only I could think wisely or rationally, even when upset." As I said earlier, we're going to be focusing on your thinking and understanding emotions over the next few sessions. I call this *problem orientation,* but it doesn't matter too much what terms we use— basically I'll be working with you on learning how to think wisely and rationally—even in the face of some very intense emotions. What is happening in the situation you describe is that when you are scared or sad, you have learned to say things to yourself, almost automatically, that you may not even be immediately aware of. These may be things you have learned to say to yourself for a long time, even as a child.

GARY.   I started thinking before, when we were talking . . . that Celia really pisses me off when she tells me that I'm overreacting—reminds me of my family and everybody else who doesn't understand me.

THERAPIST.   It's not unusual for people to develop thinking habits about the way they see problems with other people. In your case, you seem to be ready and waiting to find out that someone you want to be close to doesn't understand you. How and why this happens can be due to many different reasons, including what your parents said to you or how you were raised. The point is, some of these self-statements are not true or don't apply to every situation, and actually work against your ability to solve problems effectively for yourself.

GARY.   Okay, I can see that.

THERAPIST.   Good. We will go though a whole list of possible self-statements and assumptions that people commonly make about problems, but let me point out a few that I pick up from what you have just told me and when we go through the list later, we can see how these thoughts may be stopping you from solving problems more effectively.

Clinical Commentary

The therapist introduced problem orientation by making a relevant connection to this patient's particular thoughts and how they are creating obstacles to his own ability to cope. In this way, the introduction of problem orientation takes on less of a "lecture format" and more of an interactive teaching strategy regarding each individual patient's own difficulties and problem orientation trouble spots. All of the problem orientation training strategies that are described later are most effective when frequent examples of the patient or group of patients are provided—examples that are more relevant to each patient's own situation.

Training in Problem Orientation

As illustrated in the preceding dialogue, it is important to explain to the patient that problem orientation refers to a psychological set or framework from which people understand and deal with problems in general. It is important to underscore a *positive* orientation, which facilitates problem-solving effectiveness, versus a *negative* orientation, which inhibits problem-solving effectiveness. It is also important to communicate that both of these orientations are observed among people with similar medical conditions such as cancer. Indeed, it is a well-researched phenomenon that people with a positive orientation, as compared with a negative orientation, are usually better able to cope with stressful events in their lives and experience less psychiatric distress and resulting disorders (see chapter 2). Finally, it is important to underscore that people can learn, through practice, to have a more positive orientation.

At this point, various examples can be provided to the patient. For example, regarding Gary, as his therapist continues to discuss and define problem orientation training, examples were taken from his description of troubling incidents that led to his referral. These included intense and difficult feelings, as well as an increased desire to use drugs and alcohol. Thinking about wanting to learn ways to cope with his recent diagnosis and recognizing that cancer presents many new problems to manage were cited as examples of his adopting a realistic, but positive, orientation. On the other hand, Gary's misinterpretation of the intentions of others and wanting to use drinking to avoid problems and to numb his feelings of fear and anger were cited as examples of a negative orientation toward stressors that could thwart his problem-solving efforts.

The components of a positive problem orientation should be described in ways that are relevant for the particular patient. For Gary, these components were described in terms of learning to view his feelings as important evidence that he could benefit from focusing on his interpersonal difficulties, rather than attempting to deny, avoid, or place the blame on others for these problems. Components of a positive orientation can be reviewed with the patient by providing a handout, such as the one illustrated in Figure 5.1.

Components of a positive problem orientation include the following components:

- *Positive self-efficacy beliefs.* Perception that one can improve his or her quality of life through effective coping (i.e., problem solving) despite a prognosis of cancer.

FIGURE 5.1

COMPONENTS OF A POSITIVE PROBLEM ORIENTATION

✓ Belief that you can improve your own quality of life

✓ Belief that problems are common and normal

✓ Ability to accurately identify problems

✓ Ability to inhibit acting impulsively when confronted with a problem

The components of a positive problem orientation handout.

- *Belief that problems are inevitable.* Belief that it is common and "normal" to have a wide range of difficulties and problems throughout one's life and specifically as a function of cancer and its treatment.
- *Ability to identify problems accurately when they occur.* Use of *affective* (e.g., sadness), *cognitive* (e.g., worry), and *physical* (e.g., digestive upset) symptoms as cues that a problem exists and as a signal to begin problem-solving efforts.
- *Ability to inhibit emotional responses.* Inhibit the impulse to respond to problems emotionally by either acting impulsively or avoiding dealing with the problem.

It is important that patients begin to believe in their ability to effect positive changes in their lives. Although initial fears of disappointment and failure will serve as cues to hold onto the false belief that no positive changes can occur, the strategies aimed at altering one's problem orientation are designed to help individuals accept the risk of periodic disappointment when weighed against the benefit of greater self-efficacy and personal control. Teaching individuals to recognize problems more accurately when they occur remains a difficult therapeutic challenge because of the strong tendency of many individuals to attribute symptoms of distress either to stable characteristics (e.g., "I'm no good at coping") or to being fully dependent on the situation (e.g., "Of course I'm depressed, I have cancer"). In such cases, the goal is to develop a more balanced and realistic recognition of the problem (e.g., "My feeling depressed is evidence that having cancer is creating many new problems for me to cope with all at once"). The strategies geared to achieve this goal are detailed below and may be used in varying order, combinations, or emphases. However, all of these interventions are aimed at increasing the four components of a positive problem orientation. These strategies include the following:

- Visualization
- Taking steps from victim to survivor
- ABC method of constructive thinking
- Reversed advocacy role-play
- Identifying problems when they occur
- STOP and THINK!
- Using feelings as cues

VISUALIZATION

As a means of increasing patients' self-efficacy beliefs regarding their own problem-solving ability, the technique of *visualization* may be useful to help restructure their image of themselves from being helpless or ineffective to one of competent persons who can solve personal problems. With this strategy, the therapist's goal is to help patients create the experience of the success in their "minds eye" and vicariously experience the potential reinforcement to be gained.

This technique involves having the patient close his or her eyes and imagine that he or she has successfully solved a current problem. Even if the patient indicates that it is not possible at present, the therapist can remind him or her to try to create an imaginary scene. The instructions should include a visualization of the end point (i.e., successful resolution of the problem). It is important to convey to the patient that "It doesn't matter how you are actually able to do it—just that a difficult problem is solved." To facilitate this process, the therapist can ask, "Did you solve the problem?" "How would your life be different with this problem solved?" "How would you be feeling?" "What would you be doing?" and "How would you feel about yourself that is different than how you were feeling moments ago?" If the patient experiences difficulty imagining him- or herself solving the problem, the therapist can suggest visualizing role models (e.g., famous figures or persons whom the patient admires) solving the same or a similar problem.

As the patient begins to visualize successful resolution to a problem, it is important for the therapist to listen carefully for the positive moments that the patient reports or experiences and to reflect these statements back to the individual (e.g., "I feel relieved" or "It must feel really good to experience relief").

The central goal of this strategy is to have people create their own positive consequences to solving a difficult problem as a motivational step toward self-efficacy. Therefore, it is also important to pay close attention and actually record positive statements to recap later for patients (e.g., "It sounds like one of the benefits to increase your problem-solving skills is being able to feel more in control of your relationships and unafraid of the future"). By asking patients to describe likely positive consequences, they will provide their own intrinsic reasons why problem solving may be important and effective for them.

Clinical Case: Gary

Gary was asked to visualize a successful resolution to marital problems and anger over his wife's reported emotional distance. He was asked to picture a time in the future when the problems that he had been discussing were successfully resolved and was then requested to describe the scene that came into his mind's eye.

GARY.   We're sitting on our back patio. I'm carving wood and Celia comes outside and sits down and puts her arm around me. We're just relaxing outside and feeling peaceful.

THERAPIST.   Tell me what this feels like.

GARY.   Nice, safe . . . like I know that Celia loves me and wants to be with me.

THERAPIST.   What are you like to be with?

GARY.   I'm calm, very different than I am now. I don't explode or get angry . . . I don't have to anymore [laughs]. I'm actually more lovable . . . So it's not just Celia—everybody likes to be around me more—I even like myself better.

THERAPIST.   So you're feeling more calm, in control, and this helps the people in your life to get closer and be more supportive and helpful to you. Without any immediate concern for how you would make this happen, do you see this scene as at all possible?

GARY.   Yeah, possible, not likely, but I'd sure like to believe it's possible.

Clinical Commentary

It is interesting to note that Gary's initial focus for a successful outcome involved an image of his wife showing concern and a desire to be with him. However, as he observes the tranquility of the scene, he describes an image of himself as calmer and more in control of his own behavior. The therapist now has a working goal that Gary himself has envisioned of helping him to achieve the more peaceful state he describes in his visualization. This takes the focus off of his complaints regarding his wife and onto how he may change or learn to instrumentally obtain the reactions from others that he desires.

JOURNEY FROM VICTIM TO SURVIVOR: A TEACHING METAPHOR

This strategy provides an opportunity for an informal lecture and discussion aimed at changing a person's views of him- or herself as a patient whom cancer has attacked and victimized to a survivor who will use all strengths and wisdom to get through the experience. An example of the handout, as contained in Figure 5.2, Taking Steps From Victim to Survivor, may be used to help teach a patient how thoughts, feelings, and behavior can all be directed to increase tolerance for stressful circumstances and painful experiences in his or her life. The visual image is one of a staircase in which a "victim" is at the bottom of the stairs and a "survivor" is at the top. It is important to remember that when discussing such images, the term *survivor* refers to emotional and psychological survival rather than to a cure of cancer. Listed below is a sample presentation of this teaching metaphor. As always, the problem-solving counselor should be careful to use phrases and examples that are particularly relevant to a given patient.

> The cancer experience, including the initial symptoms, the diagnosis, the treatment decisions, and the treatments themselves, can be stressful and traumatic. Some people have described these experiences as similar to being in a war, in which the person with cancer feels like a veteran who has engaged in battle. This includes the fear of reluctant recruitment, having to

FIGURE 5.2

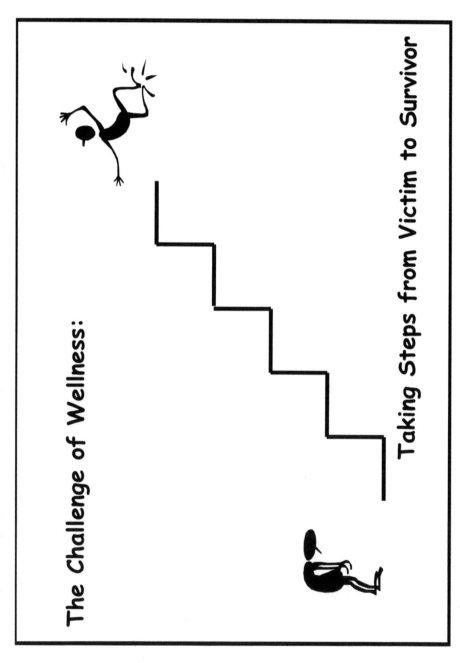

Taking steps from victim to survivor handout.

arm oneself, traveling into the unfamiliar territory of the medical culture, actually fighting the numerous and painful battles, and returning home to find out that others do not understand and often attempt to avoid talking with you about the experience.

The result of such experiences of fear, confusion, ignorance, fatigue, and rejection is evident in distressful psychological and emotional symptoms in three different areas: thoughts, feelings, and actions. Thought symptoms include worry, fear, confusion, and angry self-statements. Feelings or emoti0onal symptoms include tearfulness, embarrassment, sadness, emotional numbing, angry outbursts, and terror. Finally, action or behavioral symptoms include avoiding or denying problems, giving up, and impulsive attempts to change feelings or thoughts, such as drinking or gambling binges. [It is useful to use examples here from the individual's homework or initial interview to illustrate personally relevant examples.]

Problem-solving training provides you with weapons or survival skills that afford a way to use these three modes of functioning (thoughts, feelings, and behavior) to facilitate survival rather than experiencing disturbing obstacles to your coping efforts and quality of life. This leaves you with more resources to fight off the stress of the disease inside your body (i.e., cancer). Examples of survival thoughts include optimism that you can improve your psychological distress and the quality of your life. Survival feelings would include seeking out and focusing on pleasant experiences and emotions and using distressed feelings "as calls to action" and need for wisdom. Survival actions include asserting yourself with the medical system, seeking information, and making your own choices. A major aim of problem-solving training is to change the way you see yourself from a victim or patient with cancer to a person who can be a survivor of cancer (there is nothing very "patient" or passive about fighting cancer).

After providing the metaphor, a patient should be asked where he or she seems to be experiencing the greatest obstacles to "climbing these steps" from victim to survivor and where he or she sees him- or herself on the steps to survival at present. The obstacles should be discussed in terms of thoughts, feelings, and behavior (actions). For example, the problem-solving therapist can ask the following questions: "Where do you see yourself now on these steps?" "Are you in different places on these steps regarding your thoughts, feelings, and actions?" and "Where are you having the most difficulty walking up these steps . . . with thoughts . . . feelings . . . actions or behavior?"

We have found that the use of this teaching metaphor helps patients to translate some very complex psychological, emotional, and behavioral interactions into a conceptual framework in which their current symptoms are not viewed as failures or weaknesses but as areas in which they will need to learn and practice survival skills. The remaining problem-solving strategies can then be framed by the therapist as skills that the patients will be learning that are focused on each of the three aspects of survival. For example, the next therapy activity, which we refer to as the *ABC method of constructive thinking*, focuses on survival thoughts. Other strategies are focused specifically on feelings, actions, or behavior. For some individuals, strategies focused on any one of these areas may be more intensive because of their baseline symptoms in the area. In this way, therapy or counseling can be very individualized. As therapy continues, progress may be evaluated by having patients see themselves at different points on the staircase. For this purpose, it is useful to obtain a baseline self-rating from the patients early in treatment of their "location" on the steps from the Victim-to-Survivor handout regarding each area (i.e., thoughts, feelings, and actions). Observation of the patients' progress "up the stairs" can be shared throughout training to document improvement and reinforce patient change.

THE ABC METHOD FOR CONSTRUCTIVE THINKING

The rationale for this strategy can be explained as focusing on the thoughts that people say to themselves, their expectations of situations, and their understanding of how the world operates. Explanations frequently used in other cognitive therapies of the strong connection between how one thinks and feels (Arnkoff, 1983; Beck et al., 1979; Young & Swift, 1988) are similarly useful here when presenting a rationale to the patient. As such, the ABC model of constructive thinking is presented with the explanation that how one thinks about a situation can have a direct impact on one's emotional state. This analysis uses the following components to break down a person's internal reactions to an event.

> *A* = Activating event
> *B* = What you believe or say to yourself about A
> *C* = Emotional consequences

The therapist then personalizes the strategy by asking the individual to identify beliefs and attitudes that trigger an emotional reaction. Using an example of a current troubling experience, the therapist can use the procedure to diagnose nonconstructive or negative self-talk or thoughts that are likely to lead to unpleasant emotions. These include (a) highly evaluative words (e.g., "should" and "must"), (b) "catastrophizing" words when not pertaining to life and death circumstances (e.g., "It's awful that I was so angry, I'm terrible to be so selfish"), and (c) overgeneralizing terms (e.g., "*Nobody* can possibly understand").

The patient is directed to look at his or her own self-talk, whereby both therapist and patient can engage in separating between constructive and realistic statements (e.g., "I wish" or "I would have preferred") and nonadaptive talk (e.g., "I was stupid not to" or "I should have").

Clinical Case: Terry

Terry was experiencing significant difficulties that could be traced to a negative problem orientation. Terry had recently moved back home with her parents, and many problems involved her adjustment to a loss of independence, increased parental restriction and supervision, and dependency on her family. The problem that she selected to discuss when talking about negative thoughts and feelings involved her decrease in social activities and increased time with her parents. The transcript below provides the dialogue between Terry and her therapist regarding the use of the ABC method of constructive thinking.

TERRY.   The "A" part or activating event happened last week when my parents invited my aunt and uncle over for a barbecue, and I had really been looking forward to quietly spending the afternoon in my room, getting my new computer on-line, and getting into the Internet. My aunt and uncle seem to get along with my folks okay, but I think that they can be really boring and I didn't want to spend another Sunday with them. So I was feeling trapped and depressed.

THERAPIST.   That's a good example, Terry. Now, in order to begin to look a little more closely at your own thoughts and begin to practice more constructive thinking, let's actually begin to take apart this event, using the ABC method. The "A" was that your relatives had been invited over for a barbecue by your parents, and you preferred to do something else. Now let's list what you were actually thinking or saying to yourself about the event.

TERRY.   I feel so bad even saying it . . . I was a selfish creep.

THERAPIST.   You feel bad saying that you were feeling so badly that you cannot even report what you were thinking and feeling at the time?

TERRY.   I can report them . . . I just feel bad about it.

THERAPIST.   Explain this to me.

TERRY.   I was at first real mad and feeling sorry for myself. I was
thinking, "I don't want to spend another boring Sunday
afternoon, how come I don't get to do one thing I want to do
anymore, like work with my computer? Since I got sick, I'm
just like a little kid again." Then I started to feel real bad and
guilty. I thought "You creep, how can you be so totally selfish,
when your parents took you in, cared about you, and were
nice to you?" I started to think I really shouldn't be so picky
and I should be more willing to do what they want to do. I
should want to spend time with my aunt and uncle. Then I
started to feel really bad and wondered if maybe I got cancer
because God was punishing me for being such a selfish person.

THERAPIST.   Okay, let's list out these thoughts: "I would rather
not spend Sunday afternoon with my aunt and uncle," "I'm
just like a little kid again, because of my illness," "I am a no-
good creep and totally selfish for having these thoughts," "I
should be nicer to my parents," "I should want to spend time
with my aunt and uncle," or "I'm being punished by God
because I deserve it."

At this point the therapist and Terry went through each statement
looking for examples of evaluative language (e.g., "should" and "selfish"), catastrophizing statements ("totally selfish" and "no-good
creep"), and overgeneralizations ("punished by God because I deserve
it"). Terry was told that using a specific technique to dispute this negative self-talk and to challenge these self-statements with more constructive and truthful self-statements would be likely to help. In addition, the therapist told Terry that she would try to point out examples
of this type of negative self-talk during sessions so that she would have
much opportunity to practice challenging these thoughts. Disputing
negative self-talk consists of arguing against irrational beliefs or negative self-talk by taking an opposing or challenging viewpoint. For
example, self-statements that include words such as *should* or *ought*
need to be countered with questions such as "Why should I . . . ? Terry
gave the following answer regarding her reported belief that she
should want to spend time with her aunt and uncle.

TERRY.   There is no reason why I should want to be with my
aunt and uncle. We don't have that much in common, and
they may not particularly want to be with me either. What I'm
really experiencing here is being stuck between wanting to do
something that will be a nice way to say thank you to my
parents and wanting to do something for myself. I'm kind of
angry that I'm in this dilemma, because if I was back in my
own apartment, I wouldn't even have to make these decisions.

Challenging oneself in the use of catastrophic words while analyzing the real damage potential is an effective way to challenge these types of negative thoughts. Terry's example illustrates the point as she challenges her own thought that "I'm a selfish creep."

TERRY.   My parents enjoy their relatives, and assume that I do too. If I tell them the truth, they will probably be a bit disappointed, but won't necessarily see me as selfish, especially if I tell them that I appreciate all that they do, and if I don't try to make them give up on everything they want.

Challenging one's overgeneralizations involves objectively observing the actual validity of what is being (even silently) stated. This includes an honest assessment of what generalizations may be "fueling" particularly distressful feelings. Terry, again, provides an example.

TERRY.   I am angry that I am so dependent upon my parents and worried if I will be able to ever be on my own two feet again. At the same time, I know my parents have gone out of their way for me and I feel guilty when I get mad. Cancer is not a punishment by God. I know that. I'm exaggerating because sometimes I feel like I'm being punished, and I'm feeling quite stuck and overwhelmed. I wish that I could have my independence back.

In Terry's case, the therapist found it useful to use a handout with brief cues and instructions regarding how to identify negative self-statements and to convert such internal dialogue into more positive and realistic self-statements. We have provided an example of such a handout in Figure 5.3, Minding Your Mind: Identifying Negative Self-Talk and Converting to Positive Self-Talk. The handout provides guidelines for recognizing and challenging negative self-talk. Contained in another handout, Figure 5.4, is a list of positive self-statements that can be used to substitute for the negative self-statements. Patients are encouraged to use this list as a means of combating negative self-talk.

Clinical Commentary

Terry's ability to challenge her negative thinking was facilitated with the therapist's help. However, this scenario illustrates that by arguing against the irrational beliefs and overgeneralized self-statements, the realization that options are possible begins to emerge. For example, Terry's worries about regaining her independence can become a focus of the problem-solving treatment. Development of a plan for incremental steps toward regaining independence is likely to be more productive for Terry, as compared with silently criticizing herself for her current dependence on her parents.

FIGURE 5.3

MINDING YOUR MIND:
Identifying Negative Self-Talk and Converting to Positive Self-Talk

---

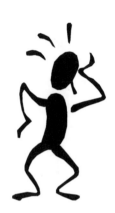

⊗ **SIGNS THAT YOU ARE USING NEGATIVE SELF-TALK**

Use of judgmental words such as "must" and "should"

Use of catastrophizing words for circumstances NOT pertaining to life and death

Overgeneralizing

➡ **METHODS FOR DISPUTING NEGATIVE SELF-TALK**

Argue against negative self-talk

Argue against "should" or "ought" with "Why should I?"

Question catastrophic words and assess **real** damage potential of situation

Challenge overgeneralizations

Use challenging POSITIVE self-statements

Minding your mind: Identifying negative self-talk and converting it to positive self-talk handout.

FIGURE 5.4

POSITIVE SELF-STATEMENTS

The following statements can be used to help you dispute negative thinking. They have actually been provided by other patients with cancer. Write those that you might find helpful on a 3" X 5" index card and carry it with you as a reminder.

I can solve this problem!
I'm okay—feeling sad is normal under these circumstances.
I can't direct the wind, but I can adjust the sails.
I don't have to please everyone.
I can replace my fears with faith.
It's okay to please myself.
There will be an end to this difficulty.
If I try, I can do it!
I can get help from _____ if I need it
It's easier, once I get started.
I just need to relax.
I can cope with this!
I can reduce my fears.
I just need to stay on track.
I can't let the worries creep in.
Prayer helps me.
I'm proud of myself!
I can hang in there!

Add your own:

List of positive self-statements handout.

REVERSED ADVOCACY ROLE-PLAY

A continuing and pervasive theme underlying all cognitive restructuring techniques is the focus on helping patients to analyze their thoughts and beliefs, as well as to test the validity and utility of these beliefs. The various schools of cognitive therapy such as Beck et al. (1979), Mahoney and Thoresen (1974), and Ellis (1985) all aim to help patients change their maladaptive beliefs and distorted perceptions of external stimuli. PST is grounded with a similar theoretical philosophy, in that an individual's unrealistic and maladaptive perceptions of problems also represent targets for change. As we have previously indicated, patients do not easily change beliefs, especially when negative emotions are aroused. To provide additional challenge to the situation, persons with chronic and life-threatening illness, such as cancer, are truly facing an extraordinary stressor. This does not mean, however, that they are not invulnerable to having irrational beliefs that require change to decrease psychological symptoms. Rather, the types of irrational thoughts are different than those dysfunctional thoughts generally associated with depressed individuals who are medically well. Thus, cognitive interventions aimed at irrational cognitions require significant adaptation for medically ill populations. For example, when working with a depressed patient, a therapist may draw attention to irrational beliefs in which the patient "makes mountains out of molehills" (i.e., overgeneralization). An example of such a belief might be as follows: "It is awful and catastrophic in my life when things do not go as planned." Using the same examples of such irrational beliefs with cancer patients could be destructive and appear disrespectful of the severity and life risk of the illness. To continue the analogy we used previously, persons with cancer are not "making mountains out of molehills" but rather are "facing and climbing mountains." The irrational beliefs on which the therapist may focus are therefore tied more to the belief that for whatever reason, the individual believes that he or she cannot climb psychological mountains. Although the concept that problems are a normal part of the cancer experience may make logical and intuitive sense to a particular patient, specific irrational and inaccurate beliefs may still be impeding the individual's ability to improve his or her quality of life.

In the reversed advocacy role-play exercise, any or all of the maladaptive irrational attitudes toward problems in the list provided below of extreme self-statements are temporarily adopted by the therapist through a role-play format. These attitudes reflect various aspects of a maladaptive problem orientation set, specifically adapted for patients with chronic illness, such as cancer. The role of the patient is to attempt to provide reasons or arguments for the statement being incorrect, maladaptive, or dysfunctional. In this manner, the patient begins to actually verbalize those aspects of a positive problem orientation. The process of identifying a more appropriate set of beliefs toward problems and providing justification for the validity of these attitudes helps the individual begin to actually personally adopt or "own" the orientation.

1. Most people do not have similar kinds of problems—no one else has difficulty coping with illness (unless they are psychologically weak).
2. All of my problems are entirely caused by having cancer. My life was perfect before having cancer, and it will be perfect again after treatment.
3. It is best to avoid facing problems or making decisions. Most problems disappear on their own.
4. The first solution that comes to mind is the best. I should always operate on instincts.
5. There is a right and a perfect solution to most problems.
6. Only someone who is experiencing the exact same problem as me can be helpful—no one else can understand.
7. People can't change. The way I am is the way I'll always be!
8. Average people cannot solve most of life's problems on their own.

We have found it useful to provide this list in written form to patients as a means of helping them to practice disputing these thoughts on their own. In addition, patients can use the list to observe their thoughts and to work with the therapist in identifying the irrational beliefs to which they are individually the most susceptible. We have provided such a handout for faulty attitudes to change—the Irrational Belief Hit List, as depicted in Figure 5.5. The list contains common irrational thoughts and provides a space for patients to write a counterstatement that challenges the inaccurate thought.

Clinical Case: Terry

In the following dialogue, the reversed advocacy role-play strategy focuses on statements from the Irrational Belief Hit List. As can be observed, Terry has strong feelings of guilt, dependency, loss, and anger.

THERAPIST.   It seems as if the way that you think very often affects your feelings. I would like to try a role-play exercise where I'll take the part of a friend of yours at work and I want you to argue with what I say. Remember, your job is to not go along with what I say, but rather to disagree with me. I'll

FIGURE 5.5

The Irrational Belief Hit List

Most people do not have problems coping with illness
Counter:

All of my problems are due to my illness
Counter:

It is better to avoid problems
Counter:

The first solution is always the best
Counter:

There is a perfect solution to each problem
Counter:

No one else can understand
Counter:

People can't change
Counter:

The irrational belief hit list: Faulty attitudes to change handout.

explain more fully after the exercise, but for now, try your best to make a valid and realistic case against any irrational, illogical, or incorrect statements that you hear, okay?

TERRY.   Okay, I'll give it a try.

THERAPIST.   I know that I seem really down lately. With all the times I cry now and think about the possibility of death, I feel like such a nutcase. Other people have cancer and seem to be a lot more courageous than me. If I have difficulty coping, it must mean that I can't cope at all and that I'm psychologically weak.

TERRY.   That's not true. A lot of people have difficulty coping with all the terrible things that we have to go through. I cry all the time. Sometimes it's real hell on earth. [Note that here Terry has begun to personalize the situation and may not be able to effectively argue. Therefore, the therapist needs to bring her back to the task.]

THERAPIST.   Remember now Terry, your job is to focus on what I am saying and argue my point. You're doing well, but try to look for a way to argue with me. Okay, let's return to the role-play. You probably don't cry as much as I do. Everyone is stronger than me. That's what makes me such a lousy patient.

TERRY.   You have no right to be so hard on yourself—look what you're going through—you didn't ask to get sick—and now you have so much more to deal with. It's hard for anyone to get sick—it may make you feel *crazy*, but you're not.

THERAPIST.   If I feel crazy, I must *be* crazy.

TERRY.   That's just an expression—it means you're upset.

THERAPIST.   So I guess I should just try to figure out a way to help myself not to be so upset?

TERRY.   Sure. You're not nuts—you're just upset.

Clinical Commentary

In this latest dialogue between Terry and her therapist, the therapist presented a theme relevant to the patient but focused on a situation that the patient could objectively appraise. The therapist's aim was to strengthen the rational attitude that this individual already had toward self-criticism. Later, when the therapist used the same strategy concerning sexual relationships and her feelings of guilt concerning her parents (both emotionally charged topics for this patient), Terry was able to engage successfully in a reversed advocacy role-play concerning these topics as well.

IDENTIFYING PROBLEMS WHEN THEY OCCUR

The purpose of this strategy is to help desensitize patients to the existence and discussion of problems and to define problems as a predictable part of cancer and its treatment, as well as a normal part of everyone's life. In addition, this focus provides the therapist with the opportunity to inquire and assess how a patient's life is different since the cancer diagnosis. Often there is change in an individual's perspective (i.e., "big" problems appear smaller compared with cancer) or a change in setting priorities (i.e., "My time with my kids is much more important than earning a big paycheck"). In addition, cancer patients often report that there are changes in the types of problems that they experience (e.g., friends may be avoidant since the cancer diagnosis or there may be a realization that previous friends or partners cannot be counted on for support). It is helpful to use a handout containing a list of problems that are common among cancer patients as a means of eliciting information about (a) the problems that a patient is currently experiencing, and (b) the problems that a patient might experience in the future because of cancer (see Figure 5.6).

If patients only identify a small number of problems, we have found it useful to ask them to develop a list of hypothetical problems for each category (i.e., "What type of problem might a person in general with cancer experience?"). Other research teams that have successfully applied problem-solving principles to individuals with chronic illness have used a problem card sort procedure (Elliot & Shewchuk, in press). This procedure involves constructing a list of common problems through either a questionnaire like the CARES or a focus group of patients and placing each problem on a separate card. Patients can be asked to sort cards into problem areas that would be most distressful to them or most disruptive to their relationships. The therapist may then emphasize these areas during training in problem orientation, as well as later during training in the rational problem-solving skills.

Clinical Case: Terry

> THERAPIST.   Looking at this list of problem areas that other people with cancer have reported experiencing, are there any areas of difficulty that pertain to your cancer experience?
>
> TERRY.   I really just hate being stuck in the house like a kid.
>
> THERAPIST.   That's a real interesting example, Terry, in that "being stuck in the house" may pertain to several types of problems on this list. For example, being stuck may be related to a physical problem, like not being able to engage in former

FIGURE 5.6

Categories of Potential Cancer-Related Problems

PHYSICAL

I have trouble walking

I have difficulty with household chores

I can't engage in recreational activities anymore

I'm losing weight

I'm having problems working

I have lots of pain

PSYCHOLOGICAL DISTRESS

I'm ashamed of the way my body looks

I worry more than ever now

Can't seem to think straight

I have problems making decisions

I have difficulty talking to my friends

Most of my friends shun me

I feel sad all the time

I have trouble sleeping

MARITAL & FAMILY

We aren't talking a lot lately

Too little affection between us

My family won't leave me alone

Change in family roles

MEDICAL INTERACTION

Can't get the information I want

Can't seem to communicate with the medical team

I don't like feeling out of control

I get nervous asking questions

SEXUAL

I lost interest in sex

Sex is difficult for me

My partner doesn't want to have sex with me anymore

List of common problems experienced by cancer patients handout.

recreational activities, stuck in the house because of wanting to avoid others, or losing friends, or it may mean something else. Can you tell me more about what this means to you?

TERRY.   It means I can't go out without my mother asking questions, now that I live with her again.

THERAPIST.   It sounds like a category of changes in relationships. In addition to adjusting to changes in relationships, what might be some other problems that you may come across during your treatment?

TERRY.   Hard to say . . . can't really think of any.

THERAPIST.   Let's look at this list that was developed by talking with many different cancer patients [takes out the list as contained in Figure 5.6]. If any of these were to happen to you, what would be most difficult or disruptive to your life?

TERRY.   I always liked my body, but right now it's hard to think about sex.

THERAPIST.   So, if you were to have difficulty in the future with the way you feel about your body or with sex, these would be particular areas of difficulty for you.

TERRY.   Yes—that would be hard.

THERAPIST.   What are the areas in which you think you may be unlikely to experience difficulties.

TERRY.   I don't have any problem with my doctor, and if she didn't tell me what I wanted to know, my family would go to another doctor—I don't see this as a big problem. I would feel really depressed if any of these psychological things happened though . . . and thinking about sex, when do you tell a guy about your surgery and your illness? That could be a real mood breaker—just thinking about it really upsets me.

Clinical Commentary

Terry sought counseling to deal with her new dependency on her family and concerns that her positive relationship with her mother had changed. She was resentful and angry over the extent of supervision under which she now lived. At first, she stated this as her sole area of difficulty. However, as problems experienced by others were shared, and as she was asked to list problems that she might experience or find difficult, other areas of concern began to emerge. Although it may be a premature conclusion at this juncture, one hypothesis concerning her earlier hesitancy to list problems is that the sexual difficulties and problems with peers may represent the more threatening and formidable problem areas.

The ultimate goal of the problem identification strategy is to develop a list of problems specific to a given patient. This list can also be completed by the patient as a homework assignment. This therapeutic strategy trains the patient to better predict and recognize the occurrence of problem situations in his or her life (problem perception). Accurate labeling of problem situations is a necessary prerequisite for future successful problem-solving efforts. Labeling a situation as a problem functions as a cue that can help inhibit the tendency to react automatically. In other words, accurate identification of a personal problem becomes a metaphoric "red light" that can be followed by the self-instruction to STOP and THINK before reacting. This strategy, described next, is often used in combination with teaching a patient to identify problems.

This technique helps to improve a patient's problem-perception skills. The therapist and patient then collaboratively predict the specific areas from the list in which the particular patient is either currently, or in the future, most likely to experience problems. Although the first alerts the patient to potential areas of difficulty that exist for persons with cancer in general, the second list provides a focus on the difficulties experienced by the patient in the here and now.

STOP AND THINK!

The STOP and THINK technique is particularly useful when it is necessary for individuals learning new ways of coping to have a cue by which they can inhibit the tendency to react automatically and often impulsively when faced with a problem. We have found it useful to have the patient visualize a stop sign or red traffic light and engage in a rehearsed self-statement to STOP and THINK when confronting a problem or experiencing a negative emotion. Familiar phrases such as "Look before you leap" may also be useful to include in the self-cuing procedure. In addition, because many individuals are familiar with the fight-or-flight theory during times of stress, some patients have accepted our rationale that when under stress, human beings have a third choice—they can "fight, flight, or think" in response to problematic internal and external experiences. This particular phrase has been useful in helping patients understand the importance of learning to *stop* the descending spiral of negative emotions and to *think* in order to understand what the problem is and then to focus attention on extending efforts to solve it. In addition, this visual red light can stop the tendency to avoid the problem, because denying that the problem exists will almost always guarantee that the problem will get worse.

The analogy or example of avoiding the possibility of a cancer diagnosis when symptoms first appear versus "early detection leads to prevention" can be explained as applicable to psychological and emotional symptoms as well.

Clinical Commentary

The importance of this strategy, as well as its effectiveness, requires continual practice. We have found it useful to provide a handout (see Figure 5.7) with the instructions to put the list of problems (developed earlier) and the STOP and THINK poster in a prominent place in the patient's home (e.g., refrigerator or bathroom mirror). In addition, the therapist can suggest that the patient carry cue cards to STOP and THINK or practice visualizing a stressful situation and immediately engage in developing a visual image of a large red stop sign.

USING FEELINGS AS CUES

Optimal problem solving requires competency in emotional regulation. Emotional regulation requires that individuals initially learn to observe objectively their affective reactions. This monitoring of one's own emotional state is a difficult and challenging skill to learn because secondary affective reactions to such phenomena (e.g., experiencing guilt after an initial or primary experience of anger) are often well learned by the time an individual reaches adulthood. A systematic approach to developing such skills includes "normalizing" the occurrence and intensity of emotions, as well as learning to capitalize on their adaptive function. As such, intense feelings become an important experience for the patient to "exploit" on behalf of his or her own psychological health. This strategy may be introduced by engaging the patient in listing, reviewing, or identifying the range of emotions one can have when experiencing a stressful problem. Note that the Taking Steps From Victim to Survivor handout (Figure 5.2) can be used for illustration purposes here once again.

Emotional arousal represents one major target for patient change. Although cognitive and behavioral spheres of assessment and therapeutic intervention represent the two other major areas of impact, patients most frequently seek treatment because of emotional symptomatology (e.g., depression and anxiety). In addition, physicians and nurses frequently refer their patients for counseling services when they observe negative and troubling emotional reactions. Common presenting complaints that are heard by counselors in such situations include experiences of anxiety, anger, sadness, pain, fear, and loss. It is also quite common for individuals to experience emotional numb-

FIGURE 5.7

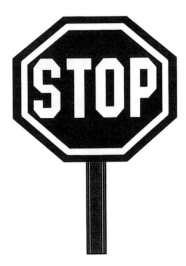

AND

THINK

STOP and THINK handout.

ness or avoidance of feelings that have become perceived of as intolerable. Whether avoiding emotions or actually experiencing significant emotional pain and distress, patients' perceptions and attributions often become negatively selective and can fuel further negative affective responses (e.g., "I get so angry at myself for feeling so down all the time"). It is not surprising that these experiences can create a downward spiral of affect and result in episodes of fatigue and a sense of hopelessness. As such, when PST is initially presented to individuals with cancer, they may react with the criticism that they already have too much burden in their life or that their only problem is cancer. Statements such as "Cure my cancer, cure my depression" or "Why should I have psychological treatment when I have a medical illness—isn't it normal to be upset?" are predictable responses that illustrate a sense of hopelessness and pessimism toward the effectiveness of any psychosocial intervention.

Creating a sufficient shift in attitudinal set so as to motivate the patient to invest additional energy often requires therapeutic skill and creativity. Therapist support and reinforcement for any independent step, especially in the initial stages of treatment, becomes a crucial element of the intervention. Validating the emotional experience of cancer and emphasizing the structure of problem solving as a means of managing these experiences while they are occurring are important to communicate to the patient.

The strategy of using feelings as cues provides patients with an understanding of how negative feelings can inhibit successful problem solving. The problem-solving handout, Steps to Wisdom (Figure 5.8), may be used to illustrate this point. Using the visual representation of two circles, in which one represents emotions and the other represents rational thinking drawn with a slight overlap, the therapist can provide a cogent rationale for the need to "facilitate one's affect and intellect working in harmony." The overlapping section is labeled as *wisdom*

FIGURE 5.8

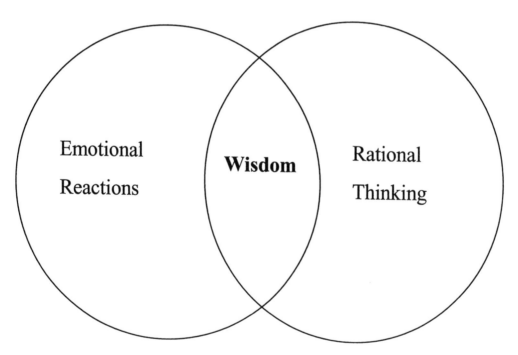

Steps to Wisdom:

Emotional

Reactions

Wisdom

Rational

Thinking

Steps to wisdom problem solving handout.

(i.e., effective problem-solving coping). The circle labeled *emotion* can be used to illustrate how negative emotions, with no rational thinking and no problem-solving efforts, can lead to additional negative emotions and negative or destructive means of expression. Rational thinking, however, without any emotions to provide clues that can guide people's rational thinking efforts, can result in a life that is empty and without passion. Conversely, when feelings are used as a clue that a problem exists, and rational thinking is used in tandem with feelings, the result is wisdom (i.e., an insightful, rational approach to understanding emotional cues).

The Understanding Emotions handout (Figure 5.9) provides a cartoon graphic that concretely reflects the complexity of examining emotions for clues. This patient handout depicts the various aspects of emotions that involve change, including *physical changes* (e.g., muscle tightness, digestive problems, and fatigue), *behavioral signs* (e.g., expressions of feelings and avoidance of feelings), changes in thoughts (e.g., repetitive thoughts and confusion), and sensory changes (e.g., the recognition that body and brain changes are taking place). For this reason, the feelings people experience when facing difficult problems may be described as "an all-encompassing emotional experience." Labeling a situation as a problem and stopping to observe and investigate one's feelings can help to inhibit the tendency to respond automatically.

Individuals who are experiencing difficulty inhibiting this tendency have found it helpful to visualize negative emotions in terms of a high mark on an emotional thermometer, as if in a red or danger zone. Much in the same way an actual thermometer alerts people to the presence of a physical problem such as an infection, an emotional thermometer alerts us to a problem that requires some resolution. As such, negative emotions are not necessarily a "bad thing," they help people to know when a problem exists and provide people with the opportunity to solve it before it gets overwhelming. When conducting training focused on using feelings as cues, it may be helpful to apply the reversed advocacy role-play strategy to specific examples of irrational thoughts people have learned concerning their emotions. Examples are given in Table 5.

Clinical Case: Gary

In the following dialogue, Gary is taught how feelings can be used as important clues to problem perception and later problem-solving attempts.

> THERAPIST.   Some of the ways people have observed their feelings as clues may be things like: noticing the experience of

FIGURE 5.9

UNDERSTANDING EMOTIONS

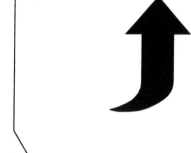

A clue to the problem!

...and a cue to STOP and think.

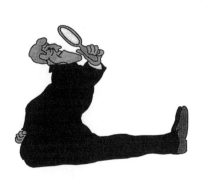

Physical Changes

Body Changes

Behavioral Signs

Changes in Thoughts

Sensory Changes

Understanding emotions handout.

TABLE 5

Irrational thoughts and counterthoughts concerning the experience of emotions

Irrational thought	Possible counterthought
I go through so many feelings—I'm a mess	All of these new feelings are cues that cancer has created many new problems for me to solve.
I just don't care anymore—Why bother?	I become exhausted when I have so many things on my mind.
I should be able to get past these emotions.	Why should I? These emotions are important indicators for me to pay attention to—they will help me identify what is important for me to change.
I can't stand it if someone gets upset with me!	I wish that this person would not overreact when I assert myself.

frustration, as though nothing you do could change anything; feeling fearful and out of control; feeling angry that you have to put up with or depend upon people; or feeling numb and distant and wanting to avoid people or situations. Some of these are actually similar to the way you described feeling when you told me about your earlier thoughts of suicide.

GARY.   I just wanted to stop the pain . . . physical, mental . . . just wanted it to stop. I could see me getting that way again if I have no hope for a cure and I know that I'm going to be in a lot of pain.

THERAPIST.   You're scared.

GARY.   Damn right, I'm scared . . . I just want to get away from everything. [Raises voice.] This problem solving is okay if the problem can be solved, like my cancer gets cured, but I don't see how it's gonna work if I don't get better!

THERAPIST.   You see what's happening here? We were noticing how scared you were—a feeling—and now you started to raise your voice and tell me problem solving is no good.

GARY.   I'm sorry. I don't want to . . .

THERAPIST.   [Interrupting.] Now you feel guilty. Let's try the technique of STOP and THINK, or stop and observe, because we have some very important feelings here—like a red light—and let's use the idea of a "feeling thermometer" to help us observe what is happening, with no judgment and no criticism, just observation.

GARY. Okay.

THERAPIST. We know that cancer is not your only problem. You have listed many problems in our previous discussion. You listed your finances, your temper and angry outbursts, your past alcohol abuse and risk of relapse, and your inability to wood carve as additional problems. Let's take a step back and look at how the emotions that you are experiencing can make a big impact on your ability to work at solving some of these problems. You told me earlier that when your wife, Celia, tried to talk to you about financial problems, you lost your temper and yelled at her, then felt guilty, wanted a drink, and thought about suicide.

GARY. Yeah, pretty messed up, isn't it?

THERAPIST. [Using Steps To Wisdom handout.] Actually, pretty predictable. If you look at this picture [pointing to emotional thoughts circle], you were reacting to your emotional experience of fear with more emotions. When no rational thinking is involved, you end up reacting to your fear with anger. Then you react to your anger with guilt. Then you react to your guilt, anger, and fear with wanting to block it out—numb it all. You know that is not likely to work since it is impossible for human beings not to feel, and so you react with thoughts of suicide—block it out entirely. Now, when we talk, you are thinking more rational thoughts [pointing to rational thinking circle], and you call your emotional reactions "messed up." You are just operating in two separate circles. Keeping them apart will create confusion and further negative feelings. However, bringing them together, to work hand in hand, will greatly enhance your problem-solving ability and overall wisdom. You have to bring the circles together, and use your first emotional experience as a clue that a problem exists—a cue to use your rational thinking. Your first emotional experience was fear. Do you see this problem going away soon? Even if your chance for remission is a good one?

GARY. No. I still have a lot to be scared of.

THERAPIST. Capture and observe that feeling of fear you had when you and Celia argued. What comes to mind?

GARY. I feel like I failed her. I'm scared she doesn't love me anymore.

THERAPIST. This is a problem that we can work on.

Clinical Commentary

In an attempt to model for Gary the STOP and THINK technique, Gary's therapist used the moment in which Gary's fear was triggered during the session and the chain of fear–anger–guilt–hopelessness was occurring in his interactions with the therapist. By imposing an atmosphere of noncritical observation and chaining back to the initial emotion, fear, the therapist was able to help Gary identify a problem for which he could apply the remaining problem-solving strategies. The cue to STOP aids in minimizing the likelihood of escalating secondary negative emotions and acting impulsively. The cue to THINK rationally involves reiterating previously practiced positive orientation statements, as well as to engage in the remainder of the problem-solving operations.

Summary

This chapter presented the therapeutic goals and strategies associated with the orientation component of PST for patients with cancer. Because the motivational sets developed during this portion of treatment significantly affect the effectiveness of later problem-solving success, a careful assessment of the therapeutic progress concerning changes in the patient's problem orientation should be conducted before continuing training in the next phase of treatment. In such a case, a problem-solving assessment measure may be readministered or examples can be given to the patient in a role-play or hypothetical format to elicit a response. Finally, there are several recommendations that can increase the likelihood of therapeutic movement during training in problem orientation. These are listed as follows:

- Do not spend too much time focusing on any one particular problem or on the person's current style of problem solving.
- Emphasize strongly the notion that negative emotions can be helpful to alert us that problems exist—it is impossible to get rid of such emotions—"We wouldn't be human without them!" The appropriate goal is to minimize the negative effects of having such emotions (e.g., increase in intensity of negative feelings leads to increase in problems).
- Emphasize the idea that not all problems can be solved (i.e., the problematic nature of the situation may be unchangeable). Rather, in certain circumstances, it is a person's reactions to the problem that may need to change (e.g., loss of a family member or anger over one's genetic predisposition to cancer).

■ Have the patient participate in exercises as much as possible. By experiencing them, he or she will begin to "own" or personally adopt a more positive orientation (e.g., by visualization). Simply telling the patient to have a "better attitude" is likely to be counterproductive. Indicate that you know and understand how difficult it may be at times.

It is important to note that continual review of the problem orientation training is an important part of future sessions in that obstacles to effective problem solving created by one's cognitive–emotional world view are likely to continue to emerge and interfere with the successful application of new coping skills throughout the training process. This review provides the therapist with frequent opportunities to provide examples, identify patient patterns that are resistant to change, and reinforce gradual patient progress.

Key Training Points

■ Teach visualization to help cancer patients "view themselves" as solving problems
■ Use journey-from-victim-to-survivor metaphor to help motivate cancer patient to engage in problem-solving attempts
■ Teach ABC method of constructive thinking to help individuals identify and then modify negative or destructive thinking patterns
■ Engage patients in reversed advocate role-playing exercises to help minimize effects of distorted thinking patterns
■ Teach patients to use feelings as cues that a problem exists
■ Teach patients to STOP and THINK

List of Suggested Handouts for Training in Problem Orientation

■ Components of a Positive Problem Orientation
■ Taking Steps From Victim to Survivor poster
■ Minding Your Mind poster
■ The Irrational Belief Hit List
■ Categories of Potential Cancer-Related Problems
■ STOP and THINK poster
■ Steps To Wisdom poster
■ Understanding Emotions poster
■ List of positive self-statements

Suggested Homework Assignments for Training in Problem Orientation

- Post the Taking Steps From Victim to Survivor handout in a very visible place (e.g., refrigerator); direct patient to look at it when feeling distressed
- Post the STOP and THINK handout in a similar place—direct patient to use it to remind him- or herself to inhibit impulsivity and to use emotions as cues that a problem exists
- Complete two Coping Attempts worksheets (Figure 3.1), including information regarding ABC model
- Bring in a brief list of problems that can serve as the focus of the remainder of PST

Group Tips

- When using the visualization exercise in a group, several variations exist. First, all group members can be asked to also close their eyes so that the person doing the visualization can feel more comfortable. Group members may either add to the person's reported positive experiences with additional positive consequences that they might foresee as an outside observer (in accordance with the visualization described) or enhance the patient's visualization by acknowledging the positive social effects. For example, if a patient in a group was visualizing herself as more assertive with her physician, other group members might add that such a successful change may make others feel more comfortable in her presence and increase their respect for the person. Another variation is to have group members engage in additional visualization themselves. If the problem situation affects more than one individual, the therapist may ask individuals to describe their positive feelings and experiences within the context of the same problem situation.
- The reversed advocacy role-play is especially conducive to group participation. Various members within a group can take turns playing the two different roles (i.e., "therapist" and "patient") while going through the entire list of "irrational beliefs." The group leader, as well as other group members, can provide feedback throughout this process. If time allows, it may also be advantageous for each group member to play both roles for each belief to gain significant practice.

Problem Definition and Formulation | 6

P *roblem definition and formulation* (PDF) represents the first of the four rational problem-solving skills. The overarching goal of training in PDF is to help a person to better understand the nature of the problem and to set realistic goals. Although the tasks involved in this aspect of the problem-solving process may be the most complex and challenging, they are also perhaps the most important. Thus, competence in this skill is crucial if the remaining problem-solving activities are to be successful. Without an accurate understanding of the problem or goal to be achieved, an individual's efforts in generating, selecting, and implementing alternative solutions are likely to be misguided and unsuccessful. On the other hand, a well-defined problem can actually facilitate one's ability to solve problems more effectively (A. Nezu & D'Zurilla, 1981a, 1981b).

Overview

When patients seek help from a mental health professional, the therapist needs to gain as thorough an understanding of their difficulties as possible, before he or she is in the best position to begin treatment. Similarly, we suggest that the problem solver needs to be able to define accurately a problem prior to thinking of possible solutions. Building on the skills learned in problem orientation, individuals should be ready to recognize problems as they occur, STOP and

THINK, and should begin to examine the nature of the problem. Often problems that seem overwhelming or too complex to manage may be reevaluated, clarified, broken into smaller problems, or redefined to represent more approachable situations. Refocusing attention away from one's emotional reaction and redirecting efforts to begin the rational problem-solving process through PDF facilitates productive thinking and minimizes the amount of energy expended feeling helpless or confused. Acquiring this new set of skills, even before completing the rest of the problem-solving training, can at times increase an individual's sense of control as it provides for a structured, systematic format in which to better understand the cause of one's distress.

In general, when people talk about daily hassles, stressors, or problems, they tend to describe them in an ambiguous and unclear manner, often providing only limited or partial information. Persons experiencing distress may seek counseling, presenting with vague and general statements, such as, "I feel out of control," "I'm afraid that I'm losing my mind," "I'm unable to cope," "I can't deal with the pressures around me anymore," "I'm becoming nasty and insensitive to those who love me," or "I'm scared of everything." Others may present what they think are very specific problems, only later to find that their chief complaints were really not the core of their distress. For example, Lydia, a 58-year-old woman diagnosed with metastatic colon cancer, initiated therapy because of worries and feelings of frustration concerning her 28-year-old daughter. She talked at length about her daughter's irresponsibility with finances, her impending move 10 hours away, and the fact that her daughter had not yet married. After several sessions of PST, Lydia was able to identify that, in fact, her "problems" were not those that she had originally mentioned. Rather, her concerns and frustrations stemmed from her fear of dying and the effects her death would have on her family. Like Lydia, people's automatic biases or subjective appraisals of problems often hinder their ability to delineate where the focus of their problem-solving efforts should be. Thus, the slogan "a problem well-defined is half solved" highlights the importance of taking the time to examine the components of a problem at its onset. Investing the time and energy to define problems, obstacles, and goals objectively often leads to an initial reduction in distress and feelings of helplessness.

Presenting the Rationale

We have found the following examples, analogies, and slogans to be helpful in emphasizing the importance underlying this process and the exercises associated with PDF training. Optimally, examples that directly relate to the patient's cancer experience, professional or personal experiences, and hobbies or recreational activities should be chosen to facilitate identification with the concepts. Depending on the patient's cognitive abilities, interests, or cultural background, different examples can be more appropriate and, thus, more effective. Once a patient accepts the rationale for this problem-solving component, he or she will be more likely to understand its applicability to stressful areas in his or her life. These following scripts are presented as possible alternative examples of how to convey the rationale of problem definition and formulation. Again, the PST counselor should use one that is particularly relevant to a given cancer patient.

PROBLEM SOLVING AS TRAVELING

Problems that remain vague and unclear become more frustrating or troublesome than may be necessary. For example, if you try to visit a friend in New York without further instructions, you may wind up in Buffalo, Rochester, or Queens. Simply looking at a map without any specific destination or guidelines would be overwhelming because there are many highways, roads, bridges, and tunnels that could lead you in an infinite number of directions. Taking many of these paths may lead you in the wrong direction, place you in dangerous territory, or cause you unnecessary time and expense. However, if you clearly define your intended destination by identifying a city, a town, and a specific address, you will be able to locate the best course of travel for your journey. You can even make your own map. Furthermore, additional details, such as landmarks, construction sites to avoid, or cross streets, will further clarify your route. Solving a problem can be thought of as successfully reaching the end of the trip. How comfortable, exciting, and educational the traveling will be depends initially on knowing where and how to reach the destination.

THE HEALTH-CARE TEAM AS PROBLEM SOLVERS

When individuals do not feel well physically, physicians, nurses, and other health-care professionals will use similar problem-solving techniques to clarify and understand the problem and to establish realistic goals for treatment. Without clearly defining the health problem, a physician may not know whether to examine the person's eye, arm, or gastrointestinal system. Does the patient need an aspirin or a tonsillectomy? Similarly, persons who are experiencing emotional distress will be able to establish appropriate and realistic goals once they learn how to pinpoint and examine what is really upsetting them.

PROBLEM SOLVING AND SPORTS

In the game of golf, if two people have comparable abilities, who is more likely to hit a hole in one—the person who identifies the flag, estimates the direction of the wind, and carefully selects the correct club, or the person who swings aimlessly without a particular hole in mind?

Training in Problem Definition and Formulation

PROBLEM DEFINITION AND FORMULATION TASKS

The following five tasks make up PDF activities:

- Seek out all available facts
- Describe the facts in clear and objective language
- Be objective—separate facts from assumptions
- Identify what makes the situation a problem
- Set realistic goals

We have found it especially helpful during PDF training to provide a handout (see Figure 6.1) containing this list to patients so that they can follow along and thus are not expected to remember a large amount of information.

GATHERING INFORMATION ABOUT THE PROBLEM

The first task in defining and formulating a problem is to gather important information about its specific nature. Cancer and its treatment present numerous novel situations for which most people do not have previous experience to draw on. Many people, however, have preconceived notions about cancer and its treatment, often derived from the media, which cannot provide individualized information. Although persons coping with a recurrence may draw on their previous bout with cancer, it may not be an accurate barometer because of potential differences in disease sites, staging, medical complications, and life circumstances. The potential danger that these frames of reference pre-

FIGURE 6.1

WHAT'S THE PROBLEM?

TASK: *Defining your problem and setting realistic goals*

REMEMBER TO:

✓ SEEK OUT ALL AVAILABLE FACTS

✓ DESCRIBE THE FACTS IN CLEAR LANGUAGE

✓ SEPARATE FACTS FROM ASSUMPTIONS

✓ IDENTIFY OBSTACLES AND CONFLICTS

✓ SET REALISTIC GOALS

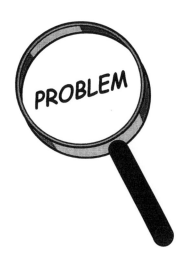

Problem definition and formulation handout.

sent is that often people draw conclusions about the nature of a problem on the basis of inaccurate or partial information. The automatic association of *death* with the word *cancer*, for example, is representative of the tendency for persons to make judgments that are based on partial information. We suggest that in most cases, "a little knowledge can be a dangerous thing," and, therefore, gathering additional information is imperative.

The problem-solving therapist should initially evaluate a patient's habituated pattern of gathering information regarding problematic situations. It is common for some people to habitually acknowledge or seek only information that supports their initial evaluation of a problem, mood state, or ineffective coping style. Specifically, depressed persons may selectively attend only to negative facts that support their feelings of hopelessness. For example, Joan, a 28-year-old woman, convinced herself that if she told her fiance that the cancer treatment might leave her infertile, he would break up with her. This was based solely on a comment that he had made in the first few months of their relationship, "Children are very important to me. When I was a camp counselor at the age of 16, I realized that I want to have many children." Without gathering more information, Joan was secretly convinced of her fiance's unwillingness to stay with her.

Anxiety may lead an impulsive person to focus on facts that suggest the need for an immediate resolution to a problem, thus disallowing time for thoughtful decision making. Consider, for example, Roger, a 39-year-old man, who described a discussion with his boss regarding an extended leave of absence related to an upcoming radiation treatment as follows: "I told him that I wasn't going to be able to lift heavy objects for quite some time. He said that he could manage the job with the workers that he had. He then asked if I would be interested in doing desk work from home while I was out . . . that would keep me involved in the project. Knowing that he said he could manage the labor without me, I had to say yes on the spot or else I might not have a job when I get better! Now I'm afraid I'm in over my head. What if I don't feel well enough to do desk work either?"

Selectively focusing only on facts that carry a positive valence can also create a biased assessment of problems, leading to unrealistic goals or ineffective decision making. Consider the following scenario described by a 60-year-old football coach, Winston, who received an allogeneic bone marrow transplant in late June. Winston had been coaching high school football for 37 years. During the season, which begins every August, Winston is responsible for the weight training and conditioning of his players, which takes place daily for 5 hours. When he asked about the likelihood of being physically able to coach during the upcoming season, his doctor replied, "It's difficult to predict exactly how you will respond to your transplant. Depending on the response to treatment, the recovery time for an allogeneic transplant typically ranges from 3 to 6 months. Some people will take longer and some *will regain their strength and energy more quickly.* If all goes well, *you could probably get involved with the team again* on a part-time basis, but I think it is unlikely that you will be able to sustain 5-hour training sessions daily." The italicized statements represent the narrow message that Winston gleaned from the conversation. He reported to his wife that the doctor told him he would be coaching again in the fall, not because he was lying, but rather, he selectively attended to what he wanted to hear.

In addition to facts that contain a positive or negative value, some facts may have no inherent emotional quality. In Winston's case, he will be required to have frequent follow-up visits with his physician after his discharge from the hospital. Although this may not be particularly upsetting for him, he would need to schedule his medical appointments at times that would not conflict with his proposed coaching schedule or his available transportation.

Gathering additional facts about a situation will help persons gain objectivity in their evaluation of a problem. Objectivity is important because persons can become aware of new perspectives from which to understand and potentially solve each difficulty that they encounter. Furthermore, collecting all of the facts about a situation avoids the mistake of making an inferential leap that could lead to further problems and confusion. For example, a patient may receive a copy of his or her blood test results and find the numbers to be lower than they had been in a prior test. However, if the patient does not have the information regarding the range of values that would be considered "normal" in each particular lab, then any conclusions drawn from the reports are likely to be misleading.

Gathering Information: Training Exercise

To facilitate efforts to gather information in an objective manner, we have found it helpful to suggest that the patient assume the role of a "detective" or an "investigative reporter." In this role, the patient's responsibility is to seek out all available information that will answer the essential questions about the "mystery" or "story" (i.e., problem) at hand. The questions to answer include: "Who?" "What?" "When?" "Where?" and "How?" If a detective needs to report this information back to headquarters, these questions would have to be answered in a thorough and objective manner to allow for an uninformed person to understand what actually happened on the basis of the details conveyed. Thus, as the questions are answered, the patient is reminded that people will only be able to see, hear, read, and agree on the validity of information only if it is a fact.

Furthermore, investigative reporters have the ethical obligation to relay all of the facts of a story as they are obtained from reliable sources. When gathering information for personal problem solving, it is also important to consider the reliability of the source of information obtained. With regard to cancer treatments, for example, a "new" intervention that is described in a trendy popular magazine, rather than in a scientific medical journal, should be regarded with some skepticism until more information can be collected.

To illustrate, we provide an example of how Gary made use of this strategy.

Clinical Case: Gary

GARY.   I got all stressed out because I was fighting with my insurance company for almost an hour on Wednesday!

THERAPIST.   Fighting with them?

GARY.   Yeah, it was a real go-around! They wanted me to go through with my transplant in some fancy hospital! I mean, easy for them to say, they're sitting behind their desks, pushing pencils, pretending like they care about anything else other than money!

THERAPIST.   Sounds like you got really angry. Were you able to put on your "detective's hat" like we talked about last week?

GARY.   Well, not at first. When they first told me that I had to go to the city for my transplant, I felt my face get hot! I guess I got kinda loud and said "What? You want me to go to the city for 5 weeks or longer?" But then I figured, I'd better keep my cool. I actually used that STOP and THINK technique. It's just that the first thing I thought of is how much I hate the city, and how I didn't want to be stuck there alone. I mean, having to go to a big-time hospital so far away from everyone. It's not like Celia has all the time in the world to drive back and forth. She has to work, and those fancy hotels in the city cost big bucks. I couldn't believe what I was hearing.

THERAPIST.   Wow. Hearing that really drummed up a lot of thoughts in your mind. You said that you were able to STOP and THINK however. That's really terrific! That will really help you when you feel yourself getting fired up. Once you did that, what happened?

GARY.   Well, I was able to pull it together. I got control of myself. That's not something I can usually do, but I did! Then I thought that I'd better get all the facts. Even if I was ticked off, I knew that Celia was going to ask me what we had to do, and I knew you'd ask me about the "detective thing!"

THERAPIST.   Well, you were right about that. It sounds like you were able to cool off a bit. What did you find out?

GARY.   What the lady said was that they know that the city hospital does the most transplants like the one that I need, and that they had some good doctors up there. The hospital near me does some transplants, but not the kind I need from someone else. That was the *why* part. She said that I'd have to go there once all the blood work and stuff was done. And she said that I could have most of the blood work and tests done at my hospital. Now I remember that's what my doc said too. So the *when* is as soon as my hospital was done with me. They would take me from my hospital to the city hospital in an ambulance, so my wife wouldn't have to drive into the city by herself that day. That was good. So I guess the *who* is the docs at both places, me, and my wife. My friends aren't in it because they won't be able to come all the way out there.

THERAPIST.   You say that your friends won't be able to visit, what facts do you have to support this? Did they tell you that?

GARY.   Well no, but it's really far. If they're like me, they hate to drive into the city. So why would they do that just to see me?

THERAPIST.   That's a good question, Gary! But I don't think I'm the best one to answer that question. Sounds like you have some more information gathering to do.

GARY.   Yeah . . . I see what you mean.

THERAPIST.   What else did you find out?

GARY.   The *how* was a big question. How could we afford to have Celia out there with me? She needs to work. She'll never be able to visit. The woman did say that there are some national services that give money to help with hotels and travel and all. But we still need money to live so that's a big thing. But really, I guess it's just that I don't want to be out there by myself!

Clinical Commentary

In this session, Gary recognized how gathering all of the information about his problem helped to contain his anger. This was due in part to the fact that he got angry on the basis of the inferential leaps that he was making and not on the facts. Because of his past negative experiences with insurance companies, Gary initially assumed that the decision for him to have the transplant in the city was without reasonable justification. On obtaining more facts, he realized his error. Furthermore, he initially targeted his dislike for the city as his "problem." As he investigated the facts, however, his problem began taking on a different definition. Rather than anger, he realized that a lot of his emotional reaction was due to the fear of the transplant and possibly dying alone.

At this point, the therapist enthusiastically reinforced Gary's effort to gather the information regarding his initial problem. However, Gary's report also revealed a need for a review of the problem orientation skills. Just as it is not uncommon for persons to seek out information in a biased manner, it is also not uncommon for people to misinterpret or distort the objective facts that they obtain. During this dialogue, Gary demonstrated some of his irrational beliefs and maladaptive self-statements that seemed to underlie his actions. Particularly, he later reported thinking that his friends would not visit him because he "wasn't worth the trip." He also selectively focused on and "catastrophized" his wife's poor financial status, which led him to believe (or in his mind "prove") that she would never be able to visit or take time off. In combination with a review of problem orientation training previously undertaken, Gary's new perspective on the definition of this particular problem was more likely to eventually produce accurate and realistic goals for a change.

Clinical Trouble-shooting

Beginning with this chapter, we offer advice specifically regarding certain difficulties that we have previously encountered when conducting PST.

▪ *Patient maintains a strong avoidance style*

It is important for the therapist to identify what obstacles the patient has encountered. For example, is the patient afraid of the information that he or she would obtain? One patient, John, stated, "I get to my doctor's office and I mean to ask questions, but then I don't!" As in this instance, conversing with physicians and health professionals can be likened to most people's encounters with auto mechanics or computer technologists if they have not had training in those fields. For many, these conversations can be intimidating, confusing, and overwhelming. A patient may, as a result, unwittingly assume a passive role in health-care decisions because he or she is too fearful to gather additional information or is afraid to challenge or possibly insult the physician. Therefore, a person coping with cancer may decide with his or her therapist that it is necessary to overcome preliminary barriers or subproblems, such as fear, before approaching larger problems. The systematic collection and use of the information gathered regarding the difficulties that the patient is experiencing during problem solving may facilitate insight and overcome preliminary problems that were not initially recognized.

■ *Patient believes that his or her situation is not a "big enough" or an "important" problem, is "not worth worrying about," or is "silly or stupid"*
It may be important to reiterate the operational definition of a problem, indicating that "a situation is a problem to the person who is experiencing it." Therefore, no problem is irrelevant or too small. As a rule, if a situation is important enough to be of concern, then it is relevant and appropriate to discuss in the counseling session.

■ *Patient believes that the problem is too pervasive, thus making it difficult to gather information*
At times, a problem may occur across situations and time points. However, it is important to help the patient concentrate on example scenarios in which the problem occurs. This will allow the therapist to assess whether the patient is overgeneralizing or catastrophizing the problem, selectively attending to negative situations, or not breaking down problems in a more manageable fashion. In addition, example situations that provide insight into the person's thoughts, feelings, and actions regarding these scenarios may help to further identify cognitive distortions or negative automatic thoughts.

DESCRIBING FACTS IN CLEAR AND UNAMBIGUOUS TERMS

This PDF task is geared to further clarify the operational definition that has begun to take form. While remembering that the goal of these initial PDF skills is to identify the overt and covert behavioral targets or emotional reactions for change, describing facts in clear and unambiguous terms helps to pinpoint why situations are problematic. Learning to use specific language in describing thoughts, feelings, and actions that are targeted for change will often decrease the perception that problems are unsurmountable. This becomes particularly true for individuals who are experiencing overwhelming emotions, such as sadness, fear, anxiety, anger, or hopelessness. When persons perceive negative emotional states that pervade across every aspect of their personal and public life, they report that their problem "equals" these emotions. However, by this point in the training process, patients should be learning that emotions in and of themselves are not the sole targets for change. In fact, feelings and emotions can be instrumental in recognizing problems as they occur. At this time, if necessary, the skill of using feelings as cues taught during the problem orientation session(s) can be reviewed once again.

Building on the task of gathering all of the facts about a problem, patients are encouraged to continue their investigation into the situations involving the painful emotions that they describe. Deciphering the *who, what, when, where,* and *how* of the patients' experienced distress will minimize the potential for misinterpretation of these events.

Clinical Case: Terry

Terry frequently recorded her feelings about living in her parents' home in her journal. Prior to learning the PDF skills, her entries described her feelings in the following way: "I feel guilty about avoiding my mom at home. It's just that we don't get along anymore like we used to." The problem-solving therapist encouraged Terry to use her journal to record her thoughts and feelings using the framework of an "investigative reporter." She agreed to document the *who, what, when, where, why,* and *how* of each specific situation in which she felt guilty or when she felt that she and her mom "were not getting along." Consider the following dialogue between Terry and her problem-solving therapist.

THERAPIST.   How was your week?

TERRY.   Well, it was okay . . . I did what we talked about. I tried to really pay attention to when my mom and I were together and I wrote a lot in my diary.

THERAPIST.   Sounds good. How did that work for you?

TERRY.   It was a lot harder to do than I thought it would be.

THERAPIST.   Okay. In what way?

TERRY.   I guess I found myself wanting to write in my diary only when I was upset. I had to really push myself to write after I was with my mom and things went okay.

THERAPIST.   Looking over what you had written, what have you learned about these situations?

TERRY.   I had to STOP and THINK several times and remember to use clear, specific words. What I realized, though, is that my mom and I still do have pleasant conversations and enjoy recreational activities together when she's not nagging me or driving me crazy.

THERAPIST.   So there are some times when you believe that you "get along." Can you use more specific or clear words to describe her "nagging" or when she's "driving you crazy?"

TERRY.   Oops! There I go again using vague language. Yeah, I wrote some of that down. I guess I just got caught up thinking about it. Basically, I get frustrated or angry when she invades my privacy or treats me like a child.

THERAPIST.   Okay. I'm still not sure what you mean when you say she "nags you," "invades your privacy," or " treats you like a child." Can you help me to better understand? Again, remember to think of the *who, what, when, where, why,* and *how.*

TERRY.   Well, for instance, on Friday I left the house while she was taking a nap. When I got home 2 hours later, she insisted on knowing where I had been and why I didn't tell her that I was leaving. Since my diagnosis, she acts like I'm so fragile. She doesn't feel like my friend anymore, I feel more like her "little girl." I mean, I only went to the library, but why does she need to know that?

THERAPIST.   Okay, now I'm starting to get a better picture. That sounds like an important question. Did you ask her why she needed to know?

TERRY.   No, I was so annoyed with her for questioning me that I didn't ask. I guess I feel like I'm 34 years old, I'm the one who knows how I'm feeling, why can't I go out without having to ask permission? But I didn't ask her that either. Then on Monday, I went shopping, and as soon as I got back she was questioning me about how do I have money to buy things I don't need? Why did I have to go to the crowded mall?

THERAPIST.   So the *who* is . . . ?

TERRY.   The *who* is my mom and me. The *what* is me living in her home again, and of course, having cancer. Also, the *what* is her asking too many questions, not respecting my privacy, and I guess being overprotective. And then my getting angry and upset. The *where* is in her home. The *when* is when I go out, or when I make plans or appointments without telling her. The *why* is, well, I guess I need to find out more about the *why.* But, I'm beginning to think it's because she's scared about "her little girl" having cancer. I actually think she feels kind of guilty herself because she had cancer a long time ago, and then I had it. But, I don't know how she feels for sure. I guess I need to find out about that.

THERAPIST.   It sounds like you do need some more information to be sure. I'm glad that makes sense to you. Can you tell me *how* these situations happen?

TERRY.   When each of these situations happened during the week, it's usually because I've made plans or decisions without talking to her. And that's been the way I've dealt with things for the past 12 or 13 years. Anyway, I would get angry because I don't think that I should have to tell her everything all of the time. That's when I would snap at her, then she'd snap back. I'd go in my room and close the door and wind up getting more upset, then feeling guilty for snapping at her in the first place. That's when I would feel like we don't get along.

THERAPIST.   You've done a really good job of trying to pinpoint the facts about your relationship with your mom. Given what you now know, how would you state your problem?

TERRY.   I guess we do get along, but the problem remains that she asks too many questions and I feel like since the cancer, she thinks she has to know everything about my life. She means well. But when these situations happen, I feel suffocated, like she is treating me like a child, and that's when I get angry and upset.

THERAPIST.   So the problem has changed somewhat?

TERRY.   Yeah. It really has. I do love my mom and that's why I feel guilty when I snap at her or get angry. I know that she loves me, and the cancer was a scare for both of us, but it's hard to deal with being so overprotected and not being as independent as I am used to. I wasn't really thinking about any of this from her point of view. It probably is really scary for her and I've been coming down on her kind of hard. I think if I ever have a daughter who has to go through this, I'd be a wreck. We haven't really talked about how *she's* doing . . .

THERAPIST.   Sounds like you're looking at this problem from a whole new angle. Your mom seems to mean a lot to you. It's understandable that you would be upset with the changes in your relationship. It also sounds like you have some more questions to get answered.

TERRY.   Yes. I think I do!

Clinical Commentary

Terry initially believed that her once treasured friendship with her mother was permanently lost and that they were not able to "get along." This ambiguous overgeneralization led her to feel more distant from her mother, as well as more upset. The use of the investigative reporter strategy led her to identify the specific conflictual situations in which she got angry with her mother. By reviewing exercises from the problem orientation sessions, the therapist helped her to recognize how her thoughts, feelings, and actions were connected in this particular problem. She realized that these events that had caused her to snap at her mother led her to feel guilty, and similarly, when she thought that her mother was "suffocating her," she felt angry and reacted negatively.

By using the investigative reporter strategy, Terry began to understand that the cancer had created a lot of changes for her and her mother that they had not discussed. Describing the facts in concrete language helped Terry gain a new perspective from which to view her problem. Terry was still saddened by the change in her relationship with her mother and her consequent angry and guilty reactions. However, she now believed that she had a better understanding of the problem and was optimistic that it could be resolved. She recognized that many positive qualities remained in her relationship with her mom. Yet, she specifically needed to address the role changes that have resulted from the diagnosis and from moving back into her parents' home.

Terry's problem needed further clarification before proceeding along in the problem-solving process. At this point in her investigation, she had obtained the facts about the situations she encountered and gained a clearer understanding of her emotional reaction to these situations. As a result, her problem definition had broadened from an emotion-focused problem to a combined emotion-focused and situation-focused problem that included her mother. It seemed likely that Terry's mother was having difficulty coping with her daughter's diagnosis, but rather than making this assumption, Terry was encouraged to continue gathering information. She intended to talk to her mother about the facts of the problem she identified. Soliciting her mother's input would help Terry to facilitate better communication between them. Discussing the problem with her would also minimize misunderstandings that have resulted in the past from the assumptions Terry made regarding her mother's behavior. Finally, Terry's definition of her problem clearly stated the situations in which she felt "overprotected" or "suffocated" by her mother. Therefore, as Terry continues her problem-solving efforts, she will have objective means by which to evaluate the outcome of her attempts to resolve this problem.

SEPARATING FACTS FROM ASSUMPTIONS

In attempting to define the nature of a problem, the patient, thus far, has learned to gather additional information and to describe these findings in clear and unambiguous terms. The next step in the PDF process is to pinpoint those elements that actually make the situation problematic, in other words, *Why* is this situation a problem? Before engaging in this assessment, the patient is trained to self-monitor his or her data collection and recording process to separate the factual information from its assumptions. Being able to discriminate facts from assumptions minimizes the likelihood that the nature of the problem is misrepresented or misunderstood because of idiosyncratic judgments, assumptions, inferences, and misinterpretations.

In some instances, problems are created on the basis of one's assumptions alone (e.g., a pseudoproblem). Such is the case with thoughts represented by "fortune telling," "what ifs," and "I just know X will happen." With each of these scenarios, people are assuming that a series of events will take place in response to a problem without having evidence to support this prediction rationally. For example, many people become distressed on the basis of the reactions they expect to get from others before the situation actually occurs. Because of people's heightened emotional state, they are less able to prevent the negative responses or to change the situation at hand and, therefore, render the situation out of their control. For example, consider a story we were told by Kenneth. Kenneth forgot to pick up his wife's prescription from the pharmacy on the way home from work. As he pulled into his driveway, he felt anxious, tense, and guilty. He thought "my wife is going to be so angry with me. Our evening is spoiled now because she can't eat dinner until I go back out and get the medication. By the time I get home, she'll be sleeping and then she's going to get nauseous from not having eaten. She's going to get sick and it's my fault." However, when Kenneth admitted to his wife that he did not purchase her medication, she replied, "Oh, that's okay. The visiting nurse will be here tomorrow and she can bring it with her. I have enough to get me through tomorrow." Kenneth had worried and aggravated himself without cause because of his fortune-telling thinking.

Defining problems on the basis of assumptions or inferences can also lead to further misguided problem-solving efforts. In Kenneth's situation, he may have decided to turn around to get his wife's medication, but that would have delayed his return home by 45 minutes. Had he done this, his wife would have been left unattended during that interval of time because her nurse's aid had left. Deciding to return for the medication on the basis of the assumption that "she would get sick" without Kenneth asking about the medication would have placed his wife at risk for injury since she would not have assistance with mobility.

Teaching persons to discriminate between facts and assumptions helps to minimize cognitive distortions, misperceptions, and inaccurate inferences. This strategy guides patients through the process of narrowing down the available information to focus on those facts that actually contribute to the problem. Thus, after gathering all of the information and describing it clearly, only that which is relevant, factual, and useful becomes the focus of strategic attention.

Separating Facts From Assumptions: Training Exercise

To introduce the concept of separating facts from assumptions, the problem-solving therapist can engage the patient in a brief exercise. It is useful to have a somewhat ambiguous photograph or picture to use as a stimulus (i.e., a magazine advertisement with the descriptive product information cutoff, a flower arrangement, or a picture in the clinician's office). The patient is asked to focus on the object or picture for about 1 minute and then to report what he or she observed. Either the therapist or the patient should record these observations for the purpose of discussion later in the session. After the patient has completed the description, the therapist provides the rationale for the exercise and for attending to the facts versus assumptions in daily problem-solving activities. On completion of this presentation, the therapist should guide the patient in reviewing the recorded observations and to practice differentiating the factual information from one's opinions, judgments, or inferences. The therapist may explain the therapeutic principle in the following manner:

> People make assumptions regularly without paying much attention to this automatic thought process. For example, if a person with poor hygiene and ripped clothing approaches someone in a high-crime-rate city, one may automatically assume that person intends harm. Further, persons may inaccurately draw the conclusion that a professional does or does not have a lot of experience on the basis of what is perceived to be his or her age. When assumptions arise in the context of a problem, the negative consequences can be significant.

In addition, the therapist can provide the patient with one of the following clinical examples that we have encountered as a means of making a point.

Clinical Examples

The Phone Call

Janet, a 38-year-old woman, former cancer patient, received a message from her physician on her answering machine requesting that she return his call regarding her laboratory reports. When she did so, he was not available and the nurse answered the phone. The nurse stated that she could not release the results to her because the doctor needed to speak with her directly. Janet hung up the phone and cried almost uncontrollably because she concluded that the cancer "must have returned if the nurse didn't tell me everything was okay!" Without knowing the standard office procedures of disclosure of information, Janet assumed that "something must be really bad if he has to tell me himself." In fact, the physician's policy was not to allow results to be released to patients from anyone other than himself so that he could address any questions the patient may have at the time. From this example, it is evident that the assumptions made by Janet created undue distress that could have been avoided. If Janet had evaluated the facts of her situation, gathered more information from the nurse, and acknowledged that she was drawing conclusions on the basis of inferences, she may have been able to respond differently to the limited information that she had.

The "Bump"

Barry, a 45-year-old man, who had recently been treated for mandibular cancer, discovered a "bump" in the back of his mouth on a Saturday afternoon. He initially panicked, believing that the cancer had returned. Although he wanted to go the hospital immediately, he did not want to call the physician on a weekend. He imagined that the doctor "would think that he was overreacting and foolish if it was a false alarm." However, having learned to STOP and THINK and to objectively separate the facts from assumptions in this situation, Barry was able to reach a rational decision about what to do. The facts were as follows: He had a bump in his mouth that was painless, his physician told him to call if he ever had any questions or concerns, he has had bumps in his mouth from agitation that have been noncancerous in the past, his last scan 2 weeks ago showed that he was "cancer free," his next appointment was in 2 weeks, and he did not have any other symptoms (e.g., bleeding or fever). On the basis of the limited factual information he had, he did not have enough evidence to suggest that the cancer had returned or that, in fact, it had not. Barry called his physician and met him at the hospital within the hour. Fortunately, Barry's bump was a noncancerous inflammation. The physician restated he was glad that Barry had called, and he should never hesitate to do so regardless of the time or day. By calling his physician, Barry minimized the negative consequences of remaining fearful or worried until his next scheduled appointment. He reported having felt in control of his emotions by recognizing which information was factual and which information was based on his own inferences.

A Wise Man Knows What He Knows and Knows What He Does Not Know

Wayne, a 26-year-old man, was becoming frustrated with his difficulty in finding a job. Because of his preexisting medical condition of cancer, several employers had indirectly asserted that Wayne may not have the strength or qualifications for the labor-intensive positions that they needed to fill. After an interview that Wayne believed was successful, he was anticipating a return call from the manager of the project for which he hoped to work. Instead, however, he received a message on his answering machine from a person in the company whose name he did not recognize. Discouraged that the project manager had not called, Wayne told his therapist, "Forget it. It's obvious that he doesn't think I can handle the job. They see 'cancer' on my medical history and they get scared off. So this guy's having one of his workers call to let me down easy with some lame excuse. I'm just not calling back. I guess it's time to move on."

The therapist lead Wayne through the process of separating the facts from the assumptions in this situation. Table 6 reflects their review of the information at hand. After a review of this information, Wayne reconsidered his decision to not return the call of the "unknown person." Wayne demonstrated the tendency of persons who have an impulsive style of approaching problems to base their decision making on information that they assume or infer to be true. In fact, when Wayne returned the call, he was greeted by the human resources representative who welcomed him to his new position and who wanted to discuss the company's benefits package with him.

By engaging in the PDF strategies, Wayne gained insight into a more salient component of this problem that also generalized across other problems that he had described during therapy. Namely, Wayne had doubts of his own self-efficacy and was generally characterized by poor self-esteem that had developed over the extended time period while in a weakened condition during his cancer treatment.

UNDERSTANDING THE NATURE OF A PROBLEM

Adopting the role of an investigative reporter or detective, the patient has thus far gathered information about the problem, recorded this information in an unambiguous and objective manner, separated the facts of the problem from unverifiable assumptions, and narrowed the definition of the problem to be more specific and focused. To continue in this role, in this next PDF task, the detective is asked to peer

TABLE 6

Wayne's facts versus assumptions

Facts	Assumptions
1. Wayne had previous experience in the type of work required for the job he was applying for.	1. "People don't care how much work you've done, if you've had cancer they still think you're sick."
2. The project manager said "you seem like a good fit for this job!"	2. "The project manager practically promised me the job."
3. Wayne was unsuccessful in gaining employment from previous interviews because the company claimed he was "not qualified." (Determined not relevant in this specific problem situation.)	3. "They made up an excuse because the company couldn't not hire me because of having had cancer."
	4. "I'm not as strong as I was before the cancer."
	5. "I didn't get the job—another rejection."
4. Wayne had been diagnosed with Hodgkin's disease 2 years ago and was now in remission. (Determined not relevant in this specific problem situation.)	6. "The project manager wimped out of telling me himself that I wasn't good enough for the job."
5. Wayne had difficulty changing health insurance companies in the past because of his preexisting medical condition. (Determined not relevant in this specific problem situation.)	7. "The project manager was having someone call to let me down easy."
	8. "I better move on and find something else."
6. The project manager did not call him.	
7. An unknown person from the company called him.	

through a magnifying glass to inspect the specific information gathered and to learn more about the situation as a whole. In most cases, an individual is able to learn to pinpoint why a situation is a problem by understanding the key factors that make situations problematic. For an individual who continues to have difficulty with identifying the nature of his or her problems, we suggest the following strategy—engaging in imagery and fantasy.

Understanding the Nature of a Problem: Training

Further investigation of why a situation is a problem for a specific individual will help to obtain a more accurate formulation of the problem. In this strategy, the *how* and *why* questions that may have previously been stated are reconsidered and compared with the goals the individual wishes to achieve. Recognizing the discrepancy between the demands of the situation and the desired outcome will highlight the obstacles and conflicts that make a situation a problem.

In tandem with adopting the view that problems are "normal and experienced by everyone," it is also important for patients to understand that the nature of problems differs among individuals. Specifically, stressful situations may be problematic in different ways for different people as a function of individually unique circumstances.

General Factors or Reasons Why a Situation May Be a Problem

There are several general factors or reasons why situations may be problems for particular individuals. These include obstacles, conflicts among goals, reduced ability to attain goals, and novelty. If appropriate, the problem-solving counselor should review these categories with the cancer patient.

Obstacles

Obstacles represent factors that hinder goal attainment. Often these may be situational in nature, such as a lack of resources or limited skills. They can also include strong emotional reactions that serve as barriers preventing individuals from goal attainment. Although emotional reactions are a part of normal responses to problems, at times, these emotions can become excessive or can appear to be unsurmountable. For instance, persons with cancer who are tremendously fearful of dying may avoid making necessary provisions for their death, such as drawing a will or explicating their wishes for advanced directives (i.e., living wills). Likewise, nervousness, fear, depression, poor self-esteem, lack of self-efficacy, anxiety, or even love for another can inhibit individuals from executing steps to reach their goals. Investigating the routes of these emotions may provide new perspectives from which to view and understand problems. Understanding the emotions that are inhibiting effective coping responses may also lead to redefining problems more accurately.

Conflicting Goals

Problems may also occur when persons have multiple goals that conflict with one another. Goals for problem resolution may be intrapersonal, interpersonal, or both. Intrapersonal goals pertain to oneself (i.e., decrease depression, increase assertiveness, and improve outlook on life). Interpersonal goals involve others, such as relationships with other people. Problem solving often becomes challenging when multiple factors must be considered to meet both interpersonal and intrapersonal goals.

For example, consider Carla, a 38-year-old woman with Stage IV breast cancer. She had become immobile and required 24-hour supervision and care. Her recently estranged husband, Eric, professionally experienced in critical care, volunteered to stay with her as one member of a support team on her rotating schedule. Carla's interpersonal and intrapersonal goals represented a discrepancy. Interpersonally, she did not want to promote further interaction with Eric, which could potentially create mixed messages and confusion concerning his role. However, she recognized that his experience in working in a rehabilitation hospital and his physical strength to lift her would relieve her anxiety and fear (intrapersonal goals) about the adequacy of her care.

Reduced Resources

Another factor that may cause a situation to become a problem for individuals is a reduction in one's ability or opportunity to attain goals. Tasks that may have been easy to accomplish prior to a diagnosis of cancer may become more complicated and may require more thought or effort to complete. Unfortunately, many people still experience discrimination in job promotions or salary increases resulting from their cancer diagnosis or sick leave. Others may have cognitive or physical limitations that reduce their ability to perform certain functions with the same agility as prior to their diagnosis (e.g., physical exercise, vigorous household chores, mathematical calculations, and extended work hours).

Novelty

Novel situations are problematic when persons are not equipped to handle them. New situations can engender a variety of reactions, including stress, fear, anxiety, uncertainty, or excitement. Without instructions or prior experience to guide oneself through new experiences, problems may arise. Persons may feel like a "stranger in a strange land" or like "a lost camper in the forest."

Having cancer involves multiple novel situations for which persons are unlikely to be adequately prepared. For example, a cancer patient scheduled for his or her first chemotherapy treatment may view this appointment as problematic and scary simply because he or she has never experienced chemotherapy before. In this situation, the patient would be encouraged to (a) gather all of the information about chemotherapy, (b) separate the factual information from the "horror stories" that he or she has heard or assumptions that he or she may be making, (c) describe the specific components of the chemotherapy that are responsible for the fear of treatment (e.g., feeling nauseous and having an injection), and (d) specify what he or she considers "successfully getting through treatment."

Ultimately, understanding the nature of problems (i.e., obstacles, discrepancies among goals, and novel situations) will provide "the compass to guide the process of subsequent problem-solving activities," such as generating alternative ways to solve them. Thus, the practice of recognizing the discrepancy between one's problems and one's goals, in combination with the other PDF skills, will increase the likelihood of successful problem resolution.

Multiple Factors

As with most real-life complex problems, it is often likely that multiple factors exist that serve to make the situation a problem, whether they are numerous obstacles, multiple conflicting goals, a variety of reduced resources, or any combination of such factors. As such, part of the task during this phase of problem solving would be to break down large problems into smaller ones. Moreover, when setting goals, it is important to delineate several subgoals or steps toward reaching larger goals. In addition, when choosing among solutions during the decision-making phase and when developing an overall solution plan, it is generally the case that multiple solution ideas need to be combined to address these multiple factors, either simultaneously or sequentially. In other words, certain parts of an overall solution plan would be geared to address certain subgoals, whereas other strategies would be included to reach other objectives.

Clinical Example: Tad

Tad was a 26-year-old man with osteosarcoma of the knee. At the time of his diagnosis, he had been working for an accounting firm for 6 months. Pleased with his performance, he had recently been led to believe that he was nearing a promotion. However, the demands of his treatment for cancer limited his physical, social, and occupational functioning substantially. His biggest concern was not to jeopardize his career path. The problem he described was one of his chief complaints that led him to seek therapy.

Tad stated his problem as follows: "My boss expects me to get as much work done during the 3-day weeks while I'm getting chemotherapy as I do when I'm here 5 days a week." He was able to validate this claim by producing several memos his boss sent to him detailing the demand for status reports of work not yet completed. Tad questioned his ability to achieve his desired outcome, "How can I keep up with my work and stop my boss from pressuring me during weeks I work part time?"

Initially, Tad had limited insight as to the reasons he was experiencing difficulty coping with his work-related responsibilities. However, the use of brainstorming strategies (see chapter 7) helped him to identify what made this situation particularly troubling for him. He identified several reasons and attempted to list them using clear and unambiguous terms: (a) accepting large projects that are difficult to complete in limited time frames (setting unrealistic intrapersonal goals and reduced opportunity to attain these goals); (b) his boss's lack of knowledge about cancer treatment and its side effects (obstacle); (c) Tad's fear of being laid off for not meeting deadlines (emotional barrier); (d) Tad's fatigue, which prevented him from working longer hours (reduced capacity to attain goals); and (e) Tad's lack of assertiveness (intrapersonal difficulty and interpersonal difficulty).

Tad initially stated that he felt more overwhelmed when he reviewed the many factors that contributed to his problem. The therapist then probed to identify which factors were potentially changeable. As a result, Tad began to focus on the many ways he could gain control of the situation, rather than worry exclusively about his current dissatisfaction. Tad became optimistic because his problem evidently had more than the two possible solutions he originally considered (i.e., taking an extended absence or eventually getting fired for not fulfilling his job). Evaluation of the discrepancies between his stated problem and his desired outcome highlighted the numerous points for potential intervention. In this way, the use of the PDF skills helps to propel patients forward in the problem-solving process.

Clinical Commentary

The therapist helped Tad to notice that his initial complaints resulted from several core themes that he began to identify across a number of problematic situations. Tad's lack of assertiveness and tendency to set unrealistically high expectations for himself were repeatedly identified as obstacles to goal attainment across several areas of his life. As therapy continued, Tad and the psychologist applied the problem-solving principles to learn more about such target behaviors and to develop a treatment plan to facilitate change.

Clinical Trouble-shooting

- *Patient has difficulty recognizing obstacles to successful goal attainment*
The use of imagery or visualization may facilitate this process. However, it may also be necessary to use many of the other problem-solving skills to define the obstacles that exist. For example, a patient may need to gather more information about the goals he or she has in order to know what obstacles exist to obtain them. For example, people who are not qualified for the type of job they would like to have may wish to enroll in college courses to gain the qualifications necessary. However, if they do not know the cost of such classes, where they are located, or the frequency with which they are offered, the obstacle that such individuals may identify is "not having enough information about the college courses," rather than specific information such as "unable to afford the cost of the college credits" or "do not have transportation to the school." Therefore, a patient may need to use problem-solving skills to overcome the obstacles before he or she can reevaluate the feasibility of the goals defined. As illustrated in the case example of Tad, guiding the patient in brainstorming, even before the rationale and training for this specific skill has actually been provided, may be instrumental in facilitating the process of identifying obstacles.

SETTING REALISTIC PROBLEM-SOLVING GOALS

Once a problem is identified, defined, and further clarified, patients are encouraged to specify their goals for resolving the problem situation. Referring back to the analogy presented in the beginning of this chapter, locating the destination of a journey on a map will ease the travel it takes to arrive there. The purpose for clearly stating and recording goals is threefold. This exercise allows individuals to (a) self-monitor their thought processes (i.e., rational thinking vs. maladaptive thinking), (b) identify the discrepancies between their defined problem and the desired change, and (c) evaluate the outcome of their problem-solving efforts in comparison to their goals.

Setting Realistic Goals: Training Exercise

When defining goals, patients are encouraged to continue the practice of using clear, specific, and unambiguous language. In attempting to specify goals for problem resolution, persons often recognize that goals may seem as complex as the initial problem. It is advisable to encourage them to break down the larger problem into its manageable component parts. Individuals may need to prioritize goals that would solve the problem by delineating short-term goals, long-term goals, and subgoals if relevant. In reality, most difficult problems will need to be addressed by identifying multiple subgoals to facilitate achievement of other goals.

For example, Terry's problem definition led her to the following question: "How can I feel comfortable dating men after having a radical mastectomy?" Recognizing the complexity of the problem, she decided to focus her initial problem-solving efforts on finding ways to accept or improve on her changes in appearance. Concurrently, she sought to increase her social support to help her with her adjustment. She specified her long-term goals to include meeting new people and reducing her anxiety in social interactions with men who show interest in dating her. By outlining her goals, Terry was able to break down the multiple components of the problem into manageable subgoals. Continuing to use the problem-solving skills, Terry first brainstormed alternative solutions to satisfy her subgoals. After having attained her subgoals, she then proceeded to apply her newly acquired problem-solving skills to reach her ultimate long-term goals.

Clinical Commentary

In delineating the goals for problem resolution, it is important for patients to understand the difference between two types of goals. Specifically, patients may engage in the problem-solving process to achieve problem-focused goals, emotion-focused goals, or both. Achieving either type of goal should ultimately aid patients in increasing their sense of control of problematic situations. Although not all problems are changeable or controllable, individuals can learn to control their reactions and responses to challenging situations.

Problem-focused goals are objectives that involve changing the nature of the situation to make it no longer problematic. Examples of problem-focused goals may include changing an existing situation in some way (e.g., increasing, decreasing, or improving certain activities or behaviors such as exercise or nutrition patterns), initiating new action or engaging in new behaviors or activities (e.g., finding a hobby or enrolling in college classes), or reducing discrepancies between goals. In the medical field, for example, oncologists have various problem-focused goals in treating persons with cancer. The physician's goal might be to remove or rid the person of the cancerous tissue, to reduce the size of the tumor, to contain the cancerous cells, or to provide palliative care.

When stressful situations are unchangeable, persons are encouraged to set realistic *emotion-focused goals*. Emotion-focused goals are objectives that involve achieving a personally acceptable way of coping with an unchangeable situation or changing one's emotional reactivity if it is maladaptive in the long term. Appropriately grieving for and accepting the death of a loved one, reducing the anticipatory nausea or anxiety that precedes chemotherapy, or controlling one's frustration and anger when caring for a colicky infant exemplifies emotion-focused goals. In addition, cancer patients with poor medical prognoses may not be able to change their medical condition, but they can change their outlook concerning the time they have remaining, improve the quality of their life, maximize or increase positive experiences, and increase their ability to cope with the unfortunate reality of their disease.

Undeniably, people with cancer experience many changes in their emotional well-being that can be manifested in feelings of depressed mood, anxiety, hopelessness, loss of control, or isolation. Patients should be instructed to use PDF strategies to further investigate and define problem situations involving emotions before setting these emotion-focused goals or assuming that the emotions themselves are problematic. As reiterated numerous times by this point in the training, emotions and feelings warrant attention but may disguise the actual problem to be solved. Therefore, therapists should explain that many problems may seem emotional at first but can actually, if more accurately defined, point to problem-focused goals.

We have found the following case example helpful to illustrate this point with patients. A 41-year-old male cancer patient, Alex, reported that he felt guilty because he did not have the energy to play baseball with his son the way he had in the past. Alex thought he had to face the guilt and somehow overcome it from within. However, when he defined the problem more clearly, Alex identified the goal of increasing other ways to have close, quality time with his son, such as reading books together.

Because of the complexity of most real-life problems, solving them often requires addressing multiple concerns, which can translate into both problem-focused and emotion-focused goals. Persons with cancer experience many physical, social, occupational, and emotional changes. These individuals are challenged to generate satisfactory alternative solutions to resolve problems and to improve their overall quality of life. Yet, by virtue of the lifestyle changes imposed by the cancer, persons also need to adjust their emotional reactions and expectations to realistically accept what they cannot control. Consider Jeannine, a 71-year-old married woman, who recently had her cancerous bladder removed. As a result of her surgery, she needed to catheterize herself every 4 hours. The procedure, and the anticipation of the procedure, invoked an anxious reaction in Jeannine. Furthermore, she had a major decrease in her pleasant activities, such as driving or going out of the house for extended time periods, because she wanted to avoid contending with her unchangeable situation.

In her case, Jeannine could not change the fact that she no longer had a bladder and now needed to drain the surgically implanted pouch. She sought therapy to reduce her anxiety about the catheterization process. Although the anxiety was interfering with her previous lifestyle, she assumed that a reduction in anxiety was the only changeable factor. What was not apparent to her before she clearly defined the problem was that much of her anxiety could be reduced by changing the nature of the situations she encountered. Thus, her goals changed to include emotion-focused goals and problem-focused goals. Problem-solving training gave her the tools to identify these multifaceted goals, which included the following: (a) reducing her anxiety about the catheterization procedure, (b) learning ways to control the sanitary condition in public bathrooms, and (c) reducing the potential embarrassment she may experience when traveling with friends. As such, when developing a comprehensive solution plan later during the problem-solving process, she would need to identify multiple strategies geared to address each of these goals.

Clinical Trouble-shooting

- *Patient has difficulty articulating goals for problem resolution*
An individual can better understand the nature of the problem if he or she is allowed to imagine or fantasize his or her desired outcome. The use of imagery or fantasy helps to articulate goals by giving the person "permission" to be creative and honest with him- or herself, regardless of what the person thinks he or she can or cannot do. This type of exercise may serve to minimize the automatic screening process (e.g., "That could never work for me" and "This idea is too ridiculous to mention") that frequently occurs in a person experiencing significant distress. When maladaptive negative self-talk interferes with problem solving at this PDF stage, a patient may not allow him- or herself to explore the plausibility of reaching his or her goals. Yet, the ideal problem resolution imagined may not be entirely unobtainable by the patient.

Getting back to Terry, as previously mentioned, she defined her problem as "How can I feel comfortable dating men after having a radical mastectomy?" When she was initially asked to describe her goals for resolving this problem, she simply restated, "To feel comfortable dating men given that I've had one breast removed." Obviously, this reiteration did not reveal new information, but provided a more focused context. The therapist explained the imagery exercise to Terry, suggesting that she allow her mind to conjure up her ideal resolution.

Terry engaged in visual imagery during her therapy session. She described her "ideal" scenario as "having dinner with a man that I am interested enough to go out with on a third or fourth date. After dinner, we go to a jazz club for drinks. I feel comfortable the whole time I'm there because the man seems interested in me and seems kind and caring. I'm able to tell him that I'm comfortable with him. He says he feels the same way. Then I tell him about having had a mastectomy and the scarring, and I do so without crying about it. He listens sympathetically and tells me that he cares about me, not the scars. And in this image, I feel good about myself and the way I look too. Later that evening, we become more intimate and the evening was enjoyable for both of us. I felt like a whole person again."

The result of Terry's visualization was twofold. First, the pleasant scenario Terry imagined motivated her to put forth more energy in her problem-solving efforts. Second, she was able to review the qualities of her imagery that she sought in resolution of her problem. Terry's goal was to figure out "How can I regain my self-confidence and adjust to my physical changes?" She also stated a secondary or long-term goal "to find new ways to meet men that are educated and mature and to feel comfortable in social situations again."

Summary

"A thorn can only be extracted if you know where it is." This quotation by Rabindranath Tagore, a nineteenth-century Indian philosopher and Nobel laureate, underscores the importance of a well-defined and conceptualized problem, as does the quotation by Georges Bernanos, an early twentieth-century French theologian and novelist, "The worst, the most corrupting lies, are problems poorly stated." In this context, a variety of strategies were delineated in this chapter geared to teach cancer patients to better define their problems. Having a well-defined problem now allows patients to learn the various brainstorming strategies to help generate multiple solution ideas. However, we strongly suggest that if a patient has difficulty with the definition-and-formulation tasks, more time should be devoted to helping him or her develop a minimum level of competency prior to going to this next phase of training. If such a patient continues to have difficulty, it may be important to "cycle back" to various orientation exercises to determine if he or she is having difficulties related to a lingering negative orientation. In addition, it is important to emphasize the notion that for most complex real-life problems, various factors exist that make the situation a problem and, therefore, require multiple strategies to address these various factors. This latter point becomes especially salient during the decision-making phase of problem solving.

Key Training Points

- Emphasize the importance of developing well-defined problems
- Help patient adopt a role (e.g., investigative reporter or detective) that facilitates the ability to seek and gather factual information
- Help patient minimize any tendency to focus on assumptions rather than on facts
- Teach patient to identify why the situation is a problem
- Train individual to delineate realistic goals (subgoals and objectives)
- Emphasize the importance of considering both problem-focused and emotion-focused goals
- Underscore the idea that most stressful problems have multiple problematic factors that need to be addressed by multiple strategies

Suggested Handouts

- Overview of PDF tasks
- PDF worksheet

Homework

- As in all of PST, assigning homework activities helps to facilitate learning and effective use of the various problem-solving skills. Figure 6.2 shows the worksheet we use in Project Genesis for PDF homework assignments. On this form, the patient is asked to record answers to the *who, what, when, where,* and *how* questions and to indicate ideas about *why* the situation is a problem. In addition, the patient is requested to delineate a realistic goal for this problem. We suggest that the patient practice PDF skills with this worksheet between training sessions by defining two problems prior to the next session.

FIGURE 6.2

PROBLEM DEFINITION AND FORMULATION

Remember to use concrete language!

Define your problem by answering the questions: WHO? WHAT? WHEN? WHERE? HOW?

What about this situation makes it a problem for you? What are the obstacles? What are the conflicts?

What are your goals? Are they realistic?

Problem definition and formulation worksheet.

Group Tips

- *Begin PDF training by providing a brief vignette of a benign non-cancer-related problem.* Each group member is then asked to record his or her perceptions of the problem described, including a definition of the problem, a possible goal for solving the problem, and any anticipated obstacles. Participants' responses may then be used for discussion and comparison among the members throughout the session to highlight the individualized nature of PDF.

- *Have participants disclose their many variations of problem definitions, goals, and obstacles to highlight the importance of these skills for effective communication.* In essence, clearly defined problems and goals are not inherently "wrong" but may not be consistent across individuals.

- *Seeking out all available facts.* The group setting permits the opportunity for valuable role-plays to facilitate learning this skill. Sample role-plays include (a) asking important questions regarding treatment, self-care, or prognosis during doctor–patient interactions; (b) inquiring about family members' reactions to changed responsibilities or emotional adjustment to the cancer diagnosis; and (c) confronting a coworker about alleged comments made regarding the patient's job performance or job status.

- *Describing facts in clear, objective terms.* Group facilitators should attempt to gain consensus or agreement from group members regarding the clarity and objectivity of defined problems discussed in session. Members should be encouraged to "fine tune" definitions and monitor each other's adherence to this rule.

- *Facts versus assumptions.* Rather than having individuals describe a picture or an object aloud as suggested in the individual treatment protocol, group members can be instructed to record their observations for 1 minute. This allows participants to formulate their own opinions and to evaluate their own habitual appraisals (i.e., facts vs. assumptions) before a group discussion ensues. In groups of six or larger, it is advisable to circulate two or three pictures for 1-minute intervals to permit each individual to see the stimulus closely. Furthermore, if some group members continue to have difficulty understanding the concepts illustrated with one example, additional examples are readily available.

- *In discussing participants' responses, the group leader can use an easel or chalk board to underline or separate factual responses from assumptions.* For each detail of the picture, group members should be encouraged to arrive at a consensus regarding classification.

- *When common assumptions are made because of fortune telling, catastrophizing, or other cognitive distortions, prompt other members to point out and label the appraisal error.*

- *Understanding why a situation is a problem.* Ask each member to provide his or her identified obstacles to the vignette introduced in the beginning of the session. Have the group discuss the relevance of the differences and similarities. After the key points to understanding why a situation is a problem have been introduced, the group facilitator should ask for an example of a problematic situation to be used for discussion. Each group member may then be encouraged to volunteer an example of one of the following as they might apply to the sample problem: (a) obstacles, (b) conflicting goals, (c) reduced resources, and (d) novelty.
- *Setting goals.* Participants may evaluate and provide feedback to others regarding the clarity, specificity, and realistic nature of defined goals. The group facilitator should draw attention to these key components of setting goals and dissuade evaluation of "good" versus "bad" goals or judging others' personal values.

Generation of Alternatives 7

Overview

I n this chapter, we continue using the metaphor of viewing problem solving as a journey. The traveler, or problem solver, having a destination to go toward (i.e., realistic problem-solving goal), is now challenged to find a variety of routes on the map to reach his or her destination. Thus, training in the second rational problem-solving skill, *generation of alternatives* (GOA), is intended to develop the patient's ability to originate a wide range of potential solutions for any problem encountered. The rationale for teaching an individual to think of a range of coping options creatively is based on the premise that the availability of a large number of alternative actions will increase the chances of eventually identifying effective solutions.

Often people expect that there is one "right" solution to a problem or that the first idea that comes to mind is the best one. However, research contradicts both of these claims (A. M. Nezu et al., 1989). Therefore, to maximize a person's ability to solve a wide range of problems, the therapist needs to convey the necessity of generating as many different options as possible through the application of brainstorming techniques.

Presenting the Rationale

To introduce the importance of GOA training, the problem-solving therapist should highlight the many benefits and purposes of using the brainstorming techniques. A sample "script" is presented in the following paragraph.

> Now that the problem at hand is well defined and we have a good idea about the goals that we want to reach, we should begin to think about various ideas to reach these goals. If we continue to think of problem solving as a journey, reaching the goals can be thought of as "getting from A to B," in other words, reaching our goals at Destination B. As in any journey, there might be several paths or roads to take to reach B. Often there are different consequences related to taking different paths—one might be longer, another might be more expensive, and yet another might be more scenic.
>
> With real-life problems, it is generally a good idea to think of multiple ways to solve the problem in order to eventually arrive at the best solution. This step of problem solving we refer to as *generating alternatives.* The task at hand now is to think of a comprehensive list of possible ideas. To accomplish this, we use a variety of *brainstorming principles.* Brainstorming helps to minimize dichotomous or black-and-white thinking. It helps to decreases one's tendency to react impulsively—if you have to think of a range of ideas, you are forced to be more reflective and planful. Brainstorming also increases one's flexibility and creativity, which improves the quality and quantity of solutions generated.
>
> The principles you will learn underlying brainstorming will teach you to discourage judging the ideas while thinking about novel solutions. This becomes particularly important when people have strong emotional reactions to problem situations. Emotions can often dominate or influence thinking such that people might rigidly think only of options that maintain their negative thoughts and feelings. When emotions do seem to become overwhelming, brainstorming can help people to get "back on track." Furthermore, engaging in brainstorming efforts redirects a person's time and energy to focus on the task of solving a problem. People concentrate on productive thinking rather than on the negative emotions that surround the problem.

Productive thinking involves confronting problems directly by creatively developing a list of possible ways to resolve the problems. This is in contrast to *nonproductive thinking*, which refers to cognitions unrelated to problem resolution, but rather to emotional distress. Consider the following differences in the reactions between Rita and Naomi, who both miss their train home from work. Both of them had dinner engagements scheduled for later in the evening. Rita chooses to focus on her negative thoughts of irresponsibility, carelessness, and unreliability, as well as negative emotions of sadness and anger at herself. She also focuses on her disappointment that the train is gone, which means that she will arrive home late, causing her to miss a dinner engagement. She continues to lament on these negative thoughts that spiral into more negative thoughts and emotions. Four hours later, Rita is still sitting at the station counting her "woes." These are the consequences of nonproductive thinking.

Alternatively, Naomi chooses to STOP and THINK rationally about her problem (i.e., "I have missed the train") and about her goal (i.e., "How can I get home as quickly as possible without ruining my evening, given that I have missed the most recent train?"). Following this path of productive thinking, Naomi attempts to generate alternative ways of solving her problem. Her partial list includes taking the next train and calling to delay her dinner date, taking a bus, taking a taxi, asking someone for a ride home, calling home and having someone pick her up and taking the next train, and going straight to the restaurant to meet her dinner date. Four hours later, we find Naomi enjoying a quiet evening with a pleasant companion who picked her up from a train stop located near the restaurant.

As in all other aspects of PST training, to enhance knowledge acquisition, we provide patients with handouts summarizing the principles and techniques of brainstorming. An example of such a GOA handout is provided in Figure 7.1.

Training in Brainstorming Principles

There are three main principles that help facilitate a person's ability to generate effective solutions to problems: (a) quantity breeds quality, (b) deferment of judgment, and (c) use strategies and tactics. In practicing brainstorming principles, patients are encouraged to be spontaneous, unreserved, and uninhibited in reporting their ideas during the session. In this environment, the creative, almost playful attitude that brainstorming engenders can also lead patients to lose track of the task. Therefore, the therapist is cautioned to help patients stay focused on the task with the purpose of the exercise in mind.

QUANTITY PRINCIPLE

The first principle, *quantity breeds quality,* encourages patients to generate as many ideas or solution options as possible. The concept of gen-

FIGURE 7.1

GENERATING ALTERNATIVE SOLUTIONS

TASK: *Think of a wide range of ideas for a solution*

USE THE BRAINSTORMING RULES:

✓ *Quantity leads to quality*
   ☞ **Make lists**
   ☞ **Combine ideas**
   ☞ **Change and modify ideas**

✓ *Don't judge any ideas until later*

✓ *Think of both strategies and tactics*

Other helpful hints:

✓ *How would your role model solve this problem?*

✓ *Use visualization*

✓ *Imagine yourself successfully solving this problem*

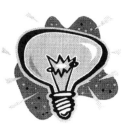

Principles of brainstorming handout.

erating numerous responses to problems, and elaborating on these responses, is supported by research findings that show that people will improve the selection of high-quality ideas by increasing the number of alternative solutions (D'Zurilla & Nezu, 1982). Research has also shown that drafting a written list of ideas, rather than composing a list of ideas in one's head, can help the patients improve both the quantity and the quality of their thinking. Recording ideas on paper keeps the problem solver focused on the task at hand and reduces repetition of ideas or "getting stuck on the same idea." Furthermore, the written results of the brainstorming exercise can be maintained for future reference and can serve as a concrete reinforcement of patients' problem-solving attempts.

Providing brief "catch phrases" can aid patients' memories during attempts to use these skills. For example, the problem-solving therapist can ask the following question: "Which store is more likely to have your size and selection, a large store or a smaller store?" Depending on the patient, this analogy can be made more specific to increase the likelihood that he or she will identify with the concepts (i.e., a diet-conscious person may have more variety in a larger market than a convenience store or a large sporting goods store will have a greater selection of tennis rackets than a smaller store).

As an aside, we have come across skeptical patients who, because they may be resistant to learning new techniques, have challenged this analogy. Consider Donnie, a 46-year-old man, who on hearing the store analogy retorted, "Well, that's not really true because when I went to buy my son's baseball pants, I checked out a few stores and the department store was more expensive than the little shop near our house! I saved 12 bucks!" In response, his therapist pointed out to him, "That's great! Yet, had you never checked out several stores, you would have never known what a great deal you got!"

DEFERMENT PRINCIPLE

The second principle, *defer judgment*, further facilitates the efficacy of brainstorming. This principle suggests that it is important for patients to record every idea that comes to their mind as a means to increase the quantity of solutions. Prematurely rejecting ideas can inhibit productive and creative thinking that often leads to potentially effective solutions. Therefore, patients are taught to refrain from evaluating solutions at this point in the problem-solving process. Reminding patients that there is no right or wrong alternative at this juncture may decrease evaluations as well.

Patients may be reluctant to disclose ideas that they believe are "silly," unrealistic, and "stupid" or that could reflect badly on them.

Therefore, the therapist needs to explain how deferring judgment actually increases one's creativity. For example, "Even if an idea seems silly or impossible initially, it may spark another related idea that is not silly or impossible." The therapist should illustrate this point during the practice exercises by offering alternatives that might be regarded as outlandish or impractical if evaluated critically. Demonstration of the ability to defer judgment and exercise freedom of thought can ease patients' flow of ideas by minimizing concern of evaluation by the therapist.

Some patients may have difficulty adhering to the deferment-of-judgment principle. These individuals may characteristically develop the "Yeah, but . . ." syndrome in response to their own alternatives or alternatives offered by the therapist. Therapists commonly hear "Yeah, *but* that won't work because . . . ," "Yeah, *but* I would never do that because . . . ," "Yeah, that sounds okay, *but* what if . . . ," or "I thought of that, *but* I didn't write it down because. . . ." Therapists may find the following analogy useful to share with such patients:

> The goal here is to come up with as many options as possible. It may help to think of the list you are putting together as a diner menu you need to prepare. On most diner menus there is a variety of options to please the tastes of children, adults, senior citizens, people who are very hungry, people who only want a snack, people who want late-night breakfast menus, desserts, or steak dinners. There may be some items on the menu that certain people might not enjoy or other items that they might not have thought of eating at a particular time of the day. But, by the fact that your restaurant offers a variety of choices, you will be more likely to satisfy your patrons. Likewise, deferring judgment about the menu of alternative solutions you create to solve your problems will increase the likelihood that you will have a variety of choices or satisfactory ideas that will meet your goals. You may not like all of the alternatives; however, there is no harm in listing them on the menu. When you engage in decision making at a later point, you can select which solutions are best suited for you.

STRATEGIES-AND-TACTICS PRINCIPLE

Learning to differentiate between *strategies and tactics*, the third principle, enhances the patients' ability to generate a multitude of solution options. *Strategies* are general courses of action people could take to solve a problem. *Tactics* are specific steps involved in putting a strategy into action. Patients are encouraged to generate as many options as possible while deferring judgment. The strategy-and-tactics principle facilitates the first two principles by providing new viewpoints from which to originate alternative solutions. Overall problem-solving efforts are likely to be less effective or productive if limited by the use of only one strategy. Therefore, the therapist should emphasize the utility of generating a wide variety of strategies and tactics rather than focusing on one or two narrow tactics or limiting oneself only to general approaches.

When patients begin to slow down in their flow of ideas while brainstorming, reviewing their written lists of solution options will enable them to classify each alternative into strategies and tactics. If they have not already done so, patients can use the strategies-and-tactics principle to help them get "unstuck" when they have difficulty generating novel ideas. Recognizing themes among the list of specific alternative solutions (tactics) and classifying these ideas under one general heading (strategies) may inspire thinking about other tactics within the same strategy. Conversely, recognizing the generality of certain solutions listed (strategies) may help to refocus brainstorming efforts to generate more specific examples.

Clinical Case: Gary

Gary developed a list of new methods of distraction that he could use to reduce his anxiety during his hospital admission in which he was scheduled to receive a bone marrow transplant. He would be confined to a small room and would be restricted from having more than two visitors at a time. Gary explained to his therapist that he had difficulty in generating many alternatives. He listed the following options: listen to music, watch soap operas, read a book, watch the news, play solitaire, talk on the phone to friends, write in a journal, look out the window, and do nothing. The therapist reviewed the list with Gary and helped him to differentiate his options into strategies and tactics. What the therapist helped Gary to notice was that several of his alternatives were very specific tactics to the same two strategies: "Activities I can do by myself" and "Look at the television." Simply by recognizing these general categories, Gary developed these ideas further (i.e., additional tactics) by thinking of what else he could do alone or could watch on television (e.g., movies provided by the hospital, rented movies, or home videos). Still, Gary had a tendency to gravitate toward one strategy.

As such, the problem-solving counselor encouraged Gary to think of additional strategies or general approaches to aid in distraction. Gary stated, "If I can do things by myself, I can also think of things I can do with others." He then managed to expand his brainstorming list by thinking of specific tactics within this new general strategy. Conversely, Gary considered his other more specific alternatives and thought of general problem-solving actions that they represented. For example, "playing solitaire" developed into the general category of "playing games." He then thought of "games to play by myself" and "games to play with others." He elaborated on these ideas by adding the following tactics: play cards with nursing staff, play cards with visitors, buy crossword puzzles, and bring the Nintendo Game Boy to the hospital. The tactic of "listening to music" was broadened to introduce the strategy of "entertain myself with my cassette recorder," which led to additional tactics of "make my own relaxation tapes, borrow my boss's time management tapes, buy or rent audio books, listen to comedians on tape, have AA sponsor tape record Alcoholics Anonymous meetings."

In this example, Gary maximized his brainstorming abilities by developing a range of different general approaches (i.e., strategies) to the problem, as well as a variety of specific, concrete actions (i.e., tactics). For Gary, periodically examining the number of strategies and tactics he listed became a fundamental skill that challenged his tendency to perseverate or get stuck on his initial ideas.

ADDITIONAL TECHNIQUES TO FACILITATE BRAINSTORMING

In addition to the three principles of brainstorming, there are several other guidelines that can facilitate the generation of new alternatives. To augment a brainstorming list that seems to be brief, people can combine ideas or modify options. When brainstorming efforts seem to lead to few strategies or tactics, the use of visualization techniques or the perspective of role models can foster creativity and productive thinking. These aids can be used by therapists to assist patients in maximizing their list of potential solutions. After the core principles of brainstorming have been practiced in session, therapists may choose to introduce these tools as a way to expand a list that was originally thought to be comprehensive. It is also appropriate to provide an overview to these additional techniques prior to beginning the brainstorming practice exercises. However, as with the introduction of any new topic or skill, caution is advised to not overwhelm the patient with too much information at one time. The techniques of using combinations, modification, models, and visualization are detailed further.

Combining Ideas

Using combinations of alternatives can be instrumental in attacking a problem from a number of perspectives. Solution alternatives may not independently achieve the desired goals; however, in combination with other ideas, the predicted outcome of the solution may change greatly. Alternatives that result from a combination of ideas may have advantages over the options already listed. For example, the combined use of surgery and chemotherapy treatment may abolish all cancer cells in a woman with a certain stage and type of breast cancer, whereas surgery alone or chemotherapy alone may be insufficient to treat the cancer. In keeping with the quantity principle and the deferment-of-judgment principle, listing the new ideas may also inspire other combinations or altogether novel ideas.

Modifying Existing Alternatives

Altering existing options is another effective means of developing new ideas. Solution options can be modified by making the alternative larger, smaller, longer, shorter, heavier, lighter, more unique, more elaborate, simpler, more complex and involving fewer people, more people, or different people. Often, alternatives can be improved on by making these adjustments; by rearranging components, patterns, or approaches; or by substituting another ingredient, process, or place.

As an example, consider Lucy, a 58-year-old woman, who started to lose her hair because of chemotherapy treatment. She had limited financial resources and could not afford to buy a wig, nor were there any donating organizations in her area. After generating alternatives, she was disappointed with her limited options of how she could improve her appearance during treatment and recovery. She was encouraged to review her list of solutions to come up with additional ideas by modifying her existing alternatives. Specifically, a friend of hers had offered to give Lucy a wig that she had used 2 years ago for the same purpose. However, the friend's wig was made of long hair that was blond in color. Lucy's natural hair was short and dark brown in color. Using the modification technique, she thought of the idea to trim her friend's wig and use dye to change the hair color to match her own. As a result, modifying an option from Lucy's original list of alternatives produced a realistic and plausible solution to her problem.

Using Models and Heroes

At times, people may have difficulty generating a list of alternatives beyond the few ineffective solutions that they have used in attempts to solve similar problems in the past. A useful strategy to overcome this difficulty, and to aid in the brainstorming process, is for patients to think of people whom they admire or respect. Recalling words of wisdom of an older family member, close friend, or mentor may be particularly helpful in generating new alternatives. If a patient is unable to think of such a person, he or she is encouraged to think of a public figure, local hero, character from a movie or book, or famous sports coach who can serve as a model (e.g., Vince Lombardi, Anthony Robbins, Ghandi, Oprah, Archbishop Desmond Tutu, or Martha Stewart).

Patients are asked to describe people whom they admire for their ability to overcome challenges or face difficult situations courageously and with success. The therapist may then guide patients' thinking by asking, "What actions would that person take if faced with the same problematic circumstances?" Considering the actions of others held in high regard, patients automatically create some distance between themselves and the problems which they have encountered. This distance, combined with a new approach to a problem, can help generate new solution options.

Visualization

Referring back to the technique described in the problem-orientation training, visualization exercises can also be used to facilitate brainstorming. Visualization aids the brainstorming process by relaxing the patient, by increasing concentration on problem solving, and by fostering creativity. People who are more inclined to react to problems impulsively may find visualization helpful in inhibiting their tendency to react to their first ideas generated in the brainstorming exercises.

The therapist should instruct patients to close their eyes and to imagine themselves successfully coping with the problem. Patients are then asked to provide detailed information about the surrounding environment and problem situation. Concentration on the five senses (i.e., what do the patients see, hear, smell, taste, and feel) to describe the scenario can elicit a more vivid image. Once the visualization can be described with detail, the therapist asks patients to describe the actions that they would take and what they would say to deal with the situation effectively. Next, patients are reminded to practice the strategies-and-tactics brainstorming principle and to incorporate the new ideas into their visualization to create new scenarios.

BRAINSTORMING TRAINING EXERCISES

Conceptually, patients may perceive brainstorming to be a simple task to accomplish. However, like many skills, application of the brainstorming principles can be more difficult than expected. Therapists can help patients overcome barriers to brainstorming by practicing the techniques in session. The brainstorming worksheet provides a model to use for recording alternatives both in session and as homework (see Figure 7.2).

FIGURE 7.2

| **GENERATING ALTERNATIVES** | *Remember to use concrete language!* |

State problem-solving goal(s) from the PDF worksheets:

Generate as many alternatives as possible–
Remember: *Quantity leads to quality!*
                   Don't judge!
                   Use both strategies and tactics!

Generation-of-alternatives worksheet handout.

During these exercises, the therapist should expect periods of silence while the patient is thinking of new alternatives. Within reasonable limits (2 or 3 minutes), silence will facilitate the brainstorming process, and, therefore, the therapist should not attempt to fill this conversational void.

As with the introduction of any new skill, it is advisable to begin practicing the application of new principles to simple, impersonal "problems" that are neutral tasks, rather than to emotionally sensitive ones. By using benign sample problems early in skill acquisition, the patient does not have the added burden of emotional factors associated with personal problems. As the individual begins to learn the skill well, more difficult and personally relevant problems can be used for practice. This is an example of the use of *shaping* as an instructional tool (see chapter 3). With regard to applying the brainstorming principles, for example, thinking of as many ways that a brick can be used, is a recommended target problem for the initial practice attempts. Additional practice exercises may include the following: "Think of as many ways possible to use a coat hanger (an egg, a broomstick, or a paper bag)."

Some individuals may believe that these simplistic or "silly" practice exercises are a waste of their time and as such may be hesitant to engage in this practice. Therapists should remind them of the importance of learning the basic skills before facing complex, emotion-laden problems: "Learning problem solving is analogous to driving a car. People usually learn to drive a car in an empty parking lot or during off-peak times on the road, rather than pulling out of their driveway onto a five-lane highway prior to gaining their confidence and competence behind the wheel." Thus, the brick exercise represents the empty parking lot. As individuals' skills increase, they will be more equipped to handle complex personal problems or the five-lane highway.

In addition to learning the skills, practice exercises are geared to overcome patients' reluctance to change habitual patterns of coping. This goal is approached by demonstrating that the conventional way of solving a problem is not the only possibility. Therapists can expect that habitual patterns of coping have developed over a lifetime. Therefore, patients may be reluctant to abandon their ineffective coping strategies. Skills learned during problem orientation (i.e., changing maladaptive thoughts) may be readdressed to help patients challenge their rationale for not trying new problem-solving methods. They may be cued to ask themselves, "How effective was my previous way of coping? If my attempt to deal with this problem was truly effective in the past, would I be encountering this level of difficulty now?"

PRACTICING WITH PERSONALLY RELEVANT PROBLEMS

After the training exercises (e.g., thinking of various uses for a brick or a coat hanger), it is imperative that the therapist encourage the patient to apply the brainstorming techniques to personally relevant problems. Similar to learning any new skill, the importance of practice, practice, and more practice cannot be overemphasized to the patient. Perhaps in-session practice of this problem-solving component may be even more important than others because creativity is without boundaries. Although there are guidelines, some patients may find the lack of structure in brainstorming more challenging, for example, than following the investigative reporter strategy. Generation of a comprehensive list of alternatives may be especially difficult if the patient's tendency is to revert back to his or her previously ineffective coping alternatives.

Clinical Case: Terry

Terry completed two PDF and GOA worksheets for homework after undergoing training in the GOA component. After considerable time spent clarifying Terry's reasons for not wanting to return to work despite her improved physical condition, she realized that she did not want to be surrounded by people who knew that she had been treated for cancer. Although she knew that her coworkers had good intentions, she did not want to continue to be characterized as a "cancer patient." Defining situations in which she felt labeled, she identified when and in which conversations she felt particularly uncomfortable. Specifically, she defined her problem as "How can I get people at work to stop telling me stories of other cancer victims?" Her list of alternative solutions, as contained in Exhibit 7.1, represents a range of strategies and tactics derived by using the brainstorming techniques and additional tools.

After the therapist scanned the completed homework sheet, the following discussion took place.

THERAPIST.   Terry, it seems that you've put a considerable amount of time into coming up with this list. I think you've done an excellent job of brainstorming a variety of solutions. What thoughts or feelings do you have about using the brainstorming skills now that you've tried it out on your own?

TERRY.   For this problem, I realized that I really put off doing the worksheet for most of the week because it really makes me angry and upset to think about the situation. Since we talked about my habit of avoiding problems, I'm starting to notice when it happens more and more. But I knew I had to work on the worksheet, especially before coming in. A lot of what we talked about in defining the problem really makes sense—I mean understanding why it upsets me and how I wish I would be treated. So, thinking about that again, I knew I just needed to sit down and start writing!

THERAPIST.   It's really important for you to be aware of when you're avoiding problems, I'm glad that you see that is

EXHIBIT 7.1

Terry's List of Potential Alternatives Completed for Homework

"How can I have people stop telling me stories of other cancer victims or cancer survivors?"

- Walk away
- Tell person I don't care to hear his or her stories
- Change topic quickly
- Don't tell people that I had cancer
- Be patient—all this will end soon—people who already know will forget as time goes on
- Be polite and listen anyway
- Use body language to show I'm not interested in listening
- Constantly move eyes
- Turn around
- Put head down
- Move around often, shift positions, and act impatient
- Ask a close friend or associate to tell others that I don't want to hear their stories
- Talk to other cancer patients to see how they handle the situation
- Tell the person how sorry I am about his or her story, but I'm doing very well thank you, and I have a great life ahead of me
- Join the breast cancer networking group at the community hospital to help me deal with this issue
- Join other support groups from various organizations and hospitals
- Talk to American Cancer Society
- Get involved with study groups that help deal with emotional issues related to concern
- Seek professional help
- Read books, brochures, and magazines on the topic
- Additional strategies added to the list during session
    Say something directly to them
    Indirectly communicate (body language, through someone else)
    Change my attitude about it
    Learn other ways to deal with this situation
    Get help to change attitude or to learn to deal with situation

becoming more apparent to you. Tell me how it was for you once you started writing—any problems, difficulties, positive or negative thoughts or feelings?

TERRY.   Actually, once I got started I got really into it. I used some of the visualization techniques to think of the different people I work with and what I could imagine them saying. I tried to think of what I would want to say or do, and what I actually might do. A couple of times I thought of things that I know I wouldn't do, but I knew I was supposed to write them down anyway. So I did. I also thought of how my best friend would deal with the situation because she always seems to know what to say in these situations. The more things I thought of, the more I felt like I had energy to get over this. You know? I mean I really started to feel like maybe the problem isn't as bad as I thought it was going to be.

THERAPIST.   It sounds like using these skills helped you to find more options to solving your problem than you thought you had?

TERRY.   It really did. And when I thought of all of the different people I could talk to about it, or places I could go for information, I felt like I wasn't so alone in this situation.

THERAPIST.   Like you could get more support in dealing with this problem.

TERRY.   Yeah. Exactly. I mean, even if I don't end up doing some of these things, I think it's good to realize that some of these choices are there if I want them to be.

THERAPIST.   That's great Terry. You did very well with this list and applying some of the different techniques that we've talked about. I'd like us to take it even a step further. Let's take another look at the different options you've come up with and see if we can even add some more! Looking at this list again, can you think of some more general categories or strategies that could summarize your list?

TERRY.   Well, I know that while I was making the list I did try to think of general things and more specific things. . . . [The therapist allows Terry to silently review her list for 2 or 3 minutes; Terry then offers the following new ideas.] Okay, I guess the overall idea might be to say something directly to the people who tell me stories, indirectly let them know how I feel about their stories, like by body language or through someone else, or something. I could change my attitude about hearing cancer victim stories. Or I could learn other ways to deal with this situation.

THERAPIST.   Anything else?

TERRY.   I think that's about all the general ideas I can think of.

THERAPIST.   You're doing a great job. How about combining ideas or modifying them? Can you think of any more using either of those strategies?

TERRY.   [Pause.] Well, I can get help to change my attitude or to learn to deal with the situation by talking to experts or joining groups or something.

THERAPIST.   Okay! Do you see how combining ideas can help to create new ideas? And by coming up with larger categories, you might be able to think of some more specific ideas?

TERRY.   Sure. Looking at this list I could probably combine a few more. Let's see. . . .

Clinical Commentary

Notice that the therapist's use of reinforcement is in response to Terry's brainstorming attempts in general. Reinforcement is essential to increase patient's confidence in his or her problem-solving abilities. However, during this exercise, it is imperative that the therapist avoids saying "good option" or similar statements. Praising specific ideas would undermine the principle of deferring judgment. Therefore, reinforcement should be restricted to the patient's overall attempts to generate a large quantity of ideas, and a variety of options, and to defer judgment during this process. It is also particularly useful for the therapist to help the patient to expand his or her list of options to prompt the use of additional techniques when he or she is new to the skill.

OTHER PROBLEM-SOLVING COMPONENTS FOR WHICH BRAINSTORMING MIGHT BE NECESSARY

Once patients begin to grasp the concept of generating alternative options and have engaged in practice exercises during the training sessions, the therapist should discuss the generalizability of the brainstorming techniques to other problem-solving components. It is important to remember that brainstorming facilitates creativity and that productive thinking helps to identify the relevance of using these techniques throughout the problem-solving process. Specifically, these principles can help patients to develop useful lists of positive self-statements to maintain a positive problem orientation. Brainstorming can aid individuals in setting goals and defining obstacles to goal attainment during the problem-definition-and-formulation process. During the process of decision making, brainstorming can be particularly helpful in predicting consequences that may arise if certain alternatives are selected as solutions. The skills taught in solution implementation and verification are also enhanced by the use of brainstorming techniques. When patients are taught to develop a monitoring system to evaluate the progress made by implementing solutions, for example, brainstorming is helpful for thinking of innovative strategies to accomplish this task. Finally, brainstorming techniques are applicable when identifying the positive and negative consequences of implementing various solutions. Thinking of a variety of pros and cons to actually carrying out a solution helps to combat the anxiety and avoidance that often accompany addressing novel or challenging situations.

Clinical Trouble-shooting

Below are some possible difficulties that the problem-solving therapist may encounter when conducting GOA training.

- *Patient continues to criticize options as they are verbalized, despite several reminders to avoid evaluating alternatives and to defer judgment.*

  In such cases, the therapist may choose to develop a monitoring system to use in session. For example, the therapist may post a chart on the wall for the course of the session to mark off each time the patient judges solution options when practicing the GOA skills. Alternatively, the therapist and patient can apply the problem-solving skills to achieve the goal "How can we reduce the likelihood that the patient will continue to criticize options before a comprehensive alternative list has been developed?" Increasing the patient's awareness of his or her tendency to make premature judgments in the problem-solving process will allow him or her to take steps to change this habit.

- *Patient claims to be "drawing a blank" and is unable to produce even one alternative option.*

  A depressed individual or a person with poor self-esteem may have particular difficulty following the deferment-of-judgment principle. These individuals may typically be highly critical of themselves and their ideas, and therefore, may have even more difficulty when asked to practice this concept aloud in session. When this problem occurs when focused on practice exercises that are impersonal or neutral in nature, it is helpful to tell the patient that "it is okay to make up an answer." Making up answers requires imagination and creativity, similar to the process of generating alternatives. However, providing the patient with the disclaimer that an idea is "made up" rather than a product of his or her own rational thought process may help to relax that patient's defensiveness. People will perceive more freedom or permission to be creative while generating alternatives because made-up responses are expected to be spontaneous and not perfect.

- *Patient is unable to generate alternatives because he or she lacks information.*

  During the brainstorming exercise, a person may experience difficulty in generating solutions because of a lack of information. If

Clinical Trouble-shooting

continued

the patient lacks information about a goal, then he or she will be unable to generate options to help achieve that goal. For example, if a person has a career goal of becoming a movie star, but lacks information regarding required training, job opportunities, location of job opportunities, salary, initial investment into portfolios, and other pertinent topics, his or her brainstorming efforts may be geared toward assumptions about the profession and training in this field. The patient should be encouraged to learn to recognize that when substantial information is lacking, the problem should be broken down into subgoals such as "How can I learn more about this profession?"

A 33-year-old woman named Vivian, who had breast cancer with metastasis to her bones, typifies the difficulty encountered in generating a comprehensive list of strategies and tactics when only partial information is acquired. Vivian shared her brainstorming homework worksheet with her therapist for which she listed options to managing cancer pain. Her alternative strategies included coping with the pain without the help of anyone, seeking the help of medical professionals, seeking the help of holistic healers, or seeking nontraditional interventions. She listed the variety of specialists within the medical field with whom she could make an appointment for pain management treatment (e.g., nurse practitioner, oncologist, psychologist, and anaesthesiologist). Tactics to her second strategy, "dealing with the pain without the help of anyone," included self-medicating by use of prescription drugs, self-medicating by use of illicit substances, decreasing physical movement by staying in bed, and using relaxation exercises and visual imagery to withstand painful intervals of time. Vivian become stuck when she attempted to generate alternative tactics to receiving help from holistic healers or nonconventional interventions. The therapist explained that at times the problem solver may need to gather more information about certain strategies to enable him or her to brainstorm options. Without having accurate and adequate information about a potential option or goal, brainstorming may be unproductive or result in haphazard guessing. Not having enough information will also limit the patient's potential to generate a variety of strategies and tactics regarding the ambiguous topic. Vivian was instructed to break down the problem into subgoals, such that she could brainstorm ideas of "gathering more information about holistic medicine and nonconventional treatments." Some of the ideas she volunteered included going to the library or searching the Internet to learn more about these treatment options, calling other people with cancer for information regarding these services, and responding to a newspaper advertisement announcing pain management benefits from hypothermia.

Summary

Creativity and *flexibility* are key words underlying the generation-of-alternatives process. To identify effective solutions eventually, we suggest that individuals should defer judgment and think of as many solution ideas as possible. Use of the various brainstorming strategies described in this chapter can often concretely demonstrate to patients that a wide variety of coping strategies and solutions are possible, thus potentially decreasing their feelings of hopelessness and despair. For example, research has indicated that a key difference in problem solving between clinically depressed and nondepressed adults is the depressed adults' inability to generate multiple solutions to stressful problems (A. M. Nezu et al., 1989). As such, having only a few options can severely limit one's ability to cope effectively. The importance of this concept is underscored in the quotation by fourteenth-century poet, Emile Chartier, "Nothing is more dangerous than an idea, when it's the only one you have."

Key Training Points

- Teach brainstorming principles: quantity breeds quality, defer judgment, and strategies and tactics
- Teach additional techniques, such as combining ideas, modifying existing ideas, using role models as examples, and visualization
- Use benign sample problems (e.g., various uses of a brick) in the beginning to facilitate early skill acquisition
- Encourage patient to practice using real-life, personally relevant problems

Suggested Handouts

- List of brainstorming principles
- GOA worksheet

Homework

- To apply the brainstorming principles to personally relevant problems and to continue practicing these skills outside of sessions, we instruct patients to first complete PDF worksheets for two new problem situations (see Figure 5.2). Using these two newly defined problems, patients should then also complete two corresponding GOA worksheets (see Figure 6.2). If previously defined problems have not been resolved, individuals should also be encouraged to derive lists of alternative solutions for these problems as additional practice.

Group Tips

- Encourage group members to minimize judgments and impulsive negative reactions to others' ideas in the group.
- Use easel or chalkboard to record alternatives—it provides a visual representation of brainstorming efforts.
- Prepare the group to expect and allow moments of silence when participants are thinking of alternatives.
- Because of time constraints and extensive modeling in a group setting, limit the brainstorming exercise to only one neutral task (i.e., brick or coat hanger) before moving on to more relevant cancer-related problems.
- Approach brainstorming exercises in an orderly fashion requesting each member to provide one alternative before soliciting additional responses from any member (i.e., sit in a circle and generate alternatives in a clockwise direction). This procedure helps to identify individuals' varied levels of skill in this problem-solving activity and requires inclusion of more passive participants.
- Continue generating alternatives in an orderly procedure (i.e., in circle) until someone gets stuck and cannot generate another alternative. Introduce the techniques to getting unstuck to assist this person and solicit the group's help when necessary.
- Review the list recorded on the easel or chalkboard and have participants recategorize ideas into strategies and tactics.

Decision
Making | 8

D *ecision making* (DM) constitutes the third rational problem-solving skill. During DM training, the therapist provides a framework for the patient to use during the process of strategically evaluating the alternative solutions derived from the problem-solving process thus far. As in each previous session, the therapist continues to demonstrate the importance and relevance of maintaining a positive problem orientation and facilitates the replacement of ineffective coping strategies, such as impulsivity or avoidance, with more effective problem-solving coping methods. The therapist's specific goal during DM training is to teach the patient how to increase the likelihood of choosing the most effective solution(s) to his or her problems. As previously defined in chapter 2, effective solutions are defined as those that not only solve the problem (e.g., overcome the obstacles or resolve the conflict) but that also maximize positive outcomes and minimize negative consequences. Essentially, DM entails the rational prediction and evaluation of consequences for each solution possibility. On the basis of this cost–benefit analysis regarding outcome, the patient is further taught to develop an overall solution plan.

Overview and Rationale

Training in PDF and GOA emphasized objective data collection, goal setting, and brainstorming methods. Throughout these procedures, the patient has been encouraged to defer judgment of solution alternatives until the systematic process of DM has been learned. At this time, the explanation for the core concepts of DM may be presented similarly to the sample provided below.

> Now that you have learned to generate a long list of possible solutions to your personal problems, it is at this point that you can begin to judge them. However, there will be a new set of rules by which to evaluate your list. These new strategies will help you to reduce the feeling of being overwhelmed and confused and to increase your feelings of control and confidence in your ability to make decisions.
>
> Remember when you were generating alternatives, you were taught to defer judgment. Now, judgment is the central activity! You will begin to evaluate the likely success of the various options and then decide which ones to carry out. People, especially when they're distressed, often wish to consider only how effective a solution might be in terms of solving the problem right now! What we're going to discuss today is a more orderly and systematic way of evaluating these different ideas in order to increase the likelihood of maximizing positive consequences and minimizing negative consequences!

REPRESENTATIVE QUOTES TO FACILITATE LEARNING

We have found the following quotes to be helpful in presenting the rationale for DM and to provoke thinking about its utility.

Second Thoughts Are Even Wiser
—Euripides

The therapist can solicit anecdotes in which the patient remembers pondering a difficult situation that resulted in a positive outcome. Gathering information regarding successful DM efforts will provide the therapist with an opportunity to reinforce skills that are consistent with those taught during this training or to make note of maladaptive thought processes that warrant attention. Furthermore, increasing the patient's introspection of successful DM will instill optimism and increase self-efficacy. The therapist should point out the benefits of drawing on past DM successes to self-motivate initiation of problem solving when difficult problems arise.

If the patient has difficulty retrieving an example of successful DM, the therapist can encourage optimism regarding the forthcoming skills. At this time, the visualization exercise learned in problem orientation training may again be appropriate to increase motivation to learn new DM skills.

He Who Hesitates Is Sometimes Saved
—Thurber

This quote can also be used with an analogy about driving. For example, it is helpful to direct the patient to consider the consequences of taking one's time and being reasonably cautious during car travel as compared with speeding, disregarding traffic signs, or not being attentive to all surrounding stimuli. Rushing usually leads to more negative consequences, regardless of the activity (i.e., driving, performing mathematical tasks, or reading directions). Although the resolution of a problem may be accomplished by haphazard or impulsive actions, the long-term results are likely to be less satisfactory.

Training in Decision Making

DEFINING THE GOALS

Once the rationale for the systematic approach to DM has been presented, the therapist should provide an operational definition for an *effective* solution. Most people think of solutions simply as actions that solve a problem. However, many *ineffective* solutions may also resolve a problem, but in the process, these ineffective solutions may create additional problems or engender unnecessary distress or complications. Therefore, it is important for the patient to redefine or expand his or her goal of choosing a plan of action not only to *solve* a problem but also to maximize positive consequences and minimize negative consequences. Without the following DM guidelines, the patient may evaluate the list of alternatives with the preconceived biases and judgments that had been deferred during brainstorming. We advocate evaluating each alternative in such a way as to suggest that even options that may seem to hold a negative valence may prove to enhance the quality of the ultimate solution chosen. To that end, the systematic approach to DM proposed here expands beyond merely selecting an alternative solution from the list previously generated. The DM skills consist of (a) identifying, predicting, and evaluating the consequences of each potential solution; (b) conducting a cost–benefit analysis of the alternatives under consideration; and (c) selecting the optimal option or combination of options to formulate an overall solution plan.

The worksheet contained in Figure 8.1 offers a framework by which to begin to understand the various aspects of effective DM.

IDENTIFYING CONSEQUENCES

When identifying the consequences of alternative solutions, the patient is encouraged to consider *personal* consequences, *social* consequences, *short-term* consequences, and *long-term* consequences. Obviously, the consequences to each alternative remain hypothetical at this stage of the problem-solving process and, therefore, cannot be verified. Thus, the patient needs to predict the outcome of implementing each alternative solution that is based on as much factual information as possible. To predict outcomes rationally, the therapist prompts the patient, when appropriate or necessary, to recall certain principles highlighted during the previous training sessions. Skills such as recognizing negative self-talk and overgeneralizations will be important to predict consequences realistically, rather than from a negative problem orientation.

PDF strategy of stating all of the information to be discussed in clear and unambiguous terms will be important to facilitate comprehension of the benefits or negative aspects of each solution. Furthermore, the investigative reporter strategy probes the patient to explore who should be considered when evaluating consequences (as defined in PDF), why a particular alternative will or will not be effective, and how it could be altered to maximize or minimize certain consequences. Thus, when identifying consequences, statements such as "It won't work" or "I wouldn't do that" are to be avoided.

Finally, brainstorming principles are also helpful to use when considering the range of consequences, rather than simply asking the sole question, "Does it solve the problem?" For example, the therapist may remind the patient that "robbing a bank" may be an alternative that meets the goal of "obtaining more money." Yet, hopefully, the patient will recognize that this solution is not optimal for a variety of reasons. Fostering creativity during the process of identifying potential consequences will improve one's DM ability. Brainstorming the effects that one's actions will have on others, in addition to oneself, will enhance perspective taking and prioritization of goals. For example, the patient who places too much emphasis on pleasing others to the detriment of him- or herself will be helped to balance these concerns appropriately. Conversely, a patient who is exclusively self-focused will learn to take into account the effects his or her actions have on others.

Initially, it is good practice for the patient to identify and predict consequences of most or all alternatives that were generated for a given problem. However, as the patient grasps the concepts in the DM

FIGURE 8.1

DECISION-MAKING WORKSHEET

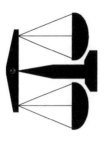

Instructions:
(1) Write the problem-solving goal
(2) Write an abbreviated form of each alternative
(3) Predict and identify consequences of implementing each alternative
(4) Evaluate each alternative using the following rating scale

Rating Scale:
+ = generally positive consequences: very likely
− = generally negative consequences: not very likely:
0 = neutral

Goal: How can I ...

Alternative	Personal Effects	Social Effects	Short-term Effects	Long-term Effects	Likelihood of Success (Will it work?)	Likelihood of Implementation (Can I do it?)

Decision-making worksheet handout.

process, the therapist may advise the patient to discard alternatives that are obviously unrelated, or contraindicative of obtaining the problem-solving goals, prior to predicting and evaluating consequences.

Personal Consequences

The individualistic nature of problem solving may be reiterated as the therapist describes how to evaluate the personal consequences of various solution alternatives. Similar to defining a problem, only the person implementing a given solution can evaluate the quality of the outcome for oneself. The personal consequences of each specific solution alternative should reflect the effects that may occur at the time of solution implementation, immediately after attempting problem resolution (short-term effects), and any resulting long-term effects. There are several factors, as outlined below, to consider when identifying and evaluating possible personal consequences. The patient is encouraged to generate a list of additional variables that may be personally relevant.

- What is the *amount of time involved* in carrying out this particular solution? Is this more or less than anticipated? Is the time frame realistic for resolving this problem?
- What is the *amount of effort required* to carry out the solution optimally?
- Is there *an emotional cost or gain* as a result of implementing this particular solution or of the potential outcome of this option?
- How will this particular solution alternative affect the person's *physical well-being?*
- Is there a *potential for personal growth* from either carrying out this solution or resolving the problem by this option?

Social Consequences

The same principles used to identify personal consequences are applicable to the identification of social consequences; namely, remembering to maintain a positive problem orientation by monitoring self-talk and physical and emotional signals of distress, using clear and unambiguous language, and brainstorming a variety of social consequences that may occur in relation to the problem-solving alternative being considered. To help the patient get started in this process, the therapist may direct him or her to think of others who have been associated with the problem as it was defined (i.e., the *who* in PDF). In general, a solution may have effects on the problem solver's (a) family, (b) friends, (c) community, and (d) on others whom the problem solver may encounter in the future. In addition, other social consequences that might be unique to a given problem should also be considered.

Short- and Long-Term Consequences

Thus far, the patient has used brainstorming guidelines to develop a list of potential consequences across personal and social domains. In reviewing this list, the patient is further asked to consider short-term consequences, or consequences that are likely to occur at the time of solution implementation, within the near future, or limited to a short period of time. Long-term consequences may include direct or indirect effects of implementing a particular solution that will exist for a longer duration of time and that will have personal or social effects in the more distant future, or over a longer period of time.

Short- and long-term consequences may represent an interaction among the personal, social, or environmental consequences (e.g., "I would feel badly if I yelled at my boss and he would be very angry, which could jeopardize my year-end bonus"). It is possible that the identified short- and long-term effects may be repetitive to those already integrated into the previous lists. However, identification of short- and long-term consequences is an important component of DM for several reasons. First, separating the short-term effects from the long-term consequences allows a patient who has an impulsive coping style to recognize that although a problem may appear to be solved when a solution is implemented, the long-term consequences may be less positive. On the other hand, a patient who is futuristic in his or her planning may overlook the negative consequences that result from using these consequences as a means to achieving an end. By separating the short- and long-term consequences of each particular alternative, the patient may better compare the positive and negative aspects of a potential solution when conducting a cost–benefit analysis later in the DM process. The therapist should also remind the patient to revisit skills from other problem-solving components as necessary to enhance his or her overall solution plan. For example, the patient may recognize that one alternative is likely to result in beneficial short-term consequences, whereas another may have more satisfying long-term consequences. Therefore, combining these alternatives, as suggested during GOA training, may result in the most effective overall solution plan if the negative consequences are few.

The importance of considering the wide range of personal and social consequences in DM is illustrated in the following comparison between two 65-year-old women, Charita and Sharon, both of whom are deciding whether or not to consent to a clinical trial for the treatment of multiple myeloma.

Charita

Charita has been widowed for 20 years. She does not have children or living relatives. She is living in a nursing home subsidized by the state where she has few friends. Her physical mobility has been progressively compromised because of non-cancer-related reasons. Personally, Charita does not want to subject herself to extended hospital stays and potential pain (short-term consequences) with no guarantee of extended survival. She is resigned to the fact that she has lived a full life and has little motivation to battle her disease with such uncertainty (long-term consequences). Although she recognizes that society and science might benefit from her participation in a clinical trial, she perceives more negative than positive consequences to this alternative. Therefore, Charita chooses to explore other options that may minimize her suffering and keep her comfortable for the duration of her life.

Sharon

Sharon has also put forth a considerable amount of thought in making her decision about the clinical trial for which she is a candidate. She knows her disease had progressed to a point in which her longevity is limited if she chooses not to accept the additional experimental treatment. With the experimental treatment, she is given a 20% chance of extending her life for another 3 years (long-term consequences). Her physician has explained the repeat hospitalization procedures and the hospital staff's ability to monitor and control pain (short-term consequences). Although she is fearful of the procedure, despite reassurance of pain control, she is compelled to accept the treatment because of factors beyond her own comfort level. Sharon has been a single mother for most of her daughter's life. Her daughter, also a single mother, lives in Sharon's home with her three children. Sharon feels a sense of responsibility to her family, both financially and emotionally. Her oldest granddaughter is engaged to be married in the near future, and the oldest grandson is going to be the first in their family to enroll in college after completion of high school in the upcoming year. Sharon hopes to be present at both of these happy occasions. If she is not able to attend, she knows that both of her grandchildren would be incredibly saddened. Even with the treatment, Sharon realizes that the negative consequences, such as the continued medical expenses, the emotional turmoil that accompanies intense treatment and uncertainty, and the necessary care she would need from her family, would all be significant burdens. However, after her overall evaluation of the personal and social consequences that may result from participation in the clinical trial, Susan decides that she and those whom she loves have more to gain than lose by her acceptance of the treatment.

EVALUATING THE CONSEQUENCES OF ALTERNATIVE SOLUTIONS AND CONDUCTING A COST–BENEFIT ANALYSIS

Value Estimates

Having predicted personal, social, and short- and long-term consequences that may result from implementing specific solutions, the patient will need a cogent way of evaluating this information. The process of evaluation is best approached by use of a simple rating scale. In our approach, we recommend that the patient should review and assign a value to each predicted consequence for each alternative. For example, a plus sign may be used to represent a positive valence, a minus sign may represent perceived negative consequences, and a zero may indicate consequences that are considered neutral (neither positive nor negative).

After a patient has assigned a rating to each consequence for an alternative under the first heading (e.g., personal consequences), he or she should designate an overall value for this alternative under this heading. For example, if three personal consequences were evaluated for one alternative and the corresponding ratings were plus, plus, and minus, the patient would characterize the personal consequences of this particular option as having more positive consequences than negative ones. On the DM sheet, then, this would be indicated by placing a large plus sign at the bottom of the box. Figure 8.2 provides for an example of how this worksheet might be completed regarding the goal of making new friends.

Next, the patient is directed to tally the pluses and minuses under the next heading, social consequences, for the same alternative. Again, the predominant number of positive, negative, or neutral consequences would indicate the valence of the social consequences predicted for that alternative. If an equal number of positive and negative consequences have been identified, it may be appropriate to assign a neutral value to the box. Similarly, if a patient had assigned two pluses and one minus to short-term effects, for example, but the intensity or the significance of the negative consequence is perceived to outweigh the positive outcomes, he or she may choose to designate a minus sign to that category. Note that caution is advised to keep the patient focused on the goal of the task, rather than becoming overly concerned with the technicalities of the process.

FIGURE 8.2

DECISION-MAKING WORKSHEET

RATING SCALE: *"+" = generally positive consequences; very likely; "–" = generally negative consequences; not very likely; "0" = neutral*

Goal: How can I ...   *Make new friends*

Alternative	Personal Effects	Social Effects	Short-term Effects	Long-term Effects	Likelihood of Success (Will it work?)	Likelihood of Implementation (Can I do it?)
1. *Join a book club*	+ Meet people with my interests – Time-consuming to read books by deadlines + Learn about new things 0 Nervous about going to first meeting alone **Overall: 0**	+ Interactive club + Structured to make getting to know people easier for everyone – Takes time away from being with my family – Late-night groups may make me less effective at work the next day **Overall: 0**	0 Nervousness 0 Awkwardness + Make time to read more 0 Need to reorganize schedule – Family will have to adapt to new schedule + Improve my mood **Overall: +**	+ May make some close friends 0 May not make any friends + May have people to get together with on weekends + Members might introduce me to their friends + Diversify reading interests 0 Family becomes a bit more independent + Feel less obligated to be home always **Overall: +**	**Overall: +**	Need to gather more information about where and when the book clubs are in the area, most likely I could do it. **Overall: ?/+**
2. *Join a health club.*						
3. *Hang-out in bars or pool halls*						
4. *Do charity work*						

Completed decision-making worksheet: Making new friends.

This simple scale is also used when evaluating two likelihood estimates (i.e., the likelihood of reaching one's goals and overcoming obstacles and the likelihood of optimal implementation). The rating scale for these likelihood estimates will reflect + (*a high likelihood/very likely*) , 0 (*neutral*), and − (*not very likely*).

Likelihood Estimates

The next step in the DM process involves identifying alternatives that are likely to solve the problem, which obviously is a major criterion contained in the operational definition of an effective solution. Identifying such options entails predictively evaluating whether the major goal(s) delineated during the PDF process would be met by implementing a given alternative. Simply put, the patient asks the following question, "Will this alternative work?" It is also important for the patient to consider the likelihood that he or she will be able to carry out the alternative optimally. Thus, the patient is essentially instructed to ask him- or herself, "Can I do it?" Other factors to consider in determining the likelihood of implementing a solution may include personal values, morals, religious, or ethical concerns. Again, the therapist should highlight the individual nature of this DM task to convey that the patient's priorities are the most important criteria to consider. Therefore, the therapist serves to help monitor the patient's approach to evaluating each option to ensure that judgments are made rationally within the context of a positive problem orientation.

When predicting the probability that a given option will successfully accomplish the problem-solving goals and will optimally be implemented, the patient is encouraged to also think in terms of the strengths and weaknesses of each option. As such, the therapist's explanation of likelihood estimates should emphasize the utility of this practice as opposed to viewing each option as good or bad or as other similar dichotomous designations. Such an approach allows the individual to review the desirable and negative aspects of each alternative and to assign an overall rating in response to each rating ("Will it work?" or "Can I do it?") according to the scale described previously. Although no solution is perfect, forming the habit of evaluating options on a continuum, rather than dichotomously, will help the patient improve his or her DM skills.

DECISION-MAKING TRAINING EXERCISES

During initial attempts to practice DM skills, the therapist should guide the patient in this process to ensure that the procedure is approached systematically. A handout of the core strategies involved in DM, as contained in Figure 8.3, is provided to the patient to facilitate the learning process.

As mentioned previously, the use of a benign example problem when learning a new skill is advisable. Such an example problem for applying DM strategies that has worked well in our experience with a variety of individuals is provided below. The therapist should supervise practice attempts to apply the DM skills to a variety of alternative solutions for a given sample problem until the patient and the therapist are satisfied with the level of competency achieved. When the patient demonstrates an adequate understanding and application of the skills with a sample problem, the therapist should encourage the patient to choose a personally relevant problem to discuss in this context.

The therapist can demonstrate the DM process by use of the following example:

> You are driving your family to a movie and are running late. You see that you are low on gas. You might be able to make it to the theater without stopping, and if you stop, you'll probably be late. On the other hand, you may not have enough gas to actually get to the theater. What do you do? One alternative is "Do not stop, keep driving to the movie." Obviously, there are many other potential solutions to this problem. For now, let's practice identifying, predicting, and evaluating hypothetical consequences that may result from implementing this one particular option.

A patient's responses to this example should be recorded on a blank DM worksheet (Figure 7.1) to help demonstrate how the cost–benefit analysis is organized. A brief period of silence is appropriate during this exercise to allow the patient to use any skills learned previously (i.e., visualization and brainstorming) to aid in the process of identifying and predicting consequences. The therapist may first offer a few example consequences to model the approach to DM. Next, the patient can be prompted to generate additional consequences. In our experience, patients have given the following responses.

1. *What are the possible personal effects of not stopping for gas?* Anxiety while driving, exhaustion from walking if we run out of gas, feel badly for disappointing family and getting them stuck, feel angry with myself for not stopping earlier.
2. *What are the possible social effects?* Family would be upset about not seeing movie, family would be upset about breaking down, family would be happy if we made it to the movies on time, everyone would have to walk a distance or be cramped in the car.
3. *What are the possible short-term effects?* Not getting to the movie at all if the car runs out of gas, have to walk for gas or be

FIGURE 8.3

DECISION MAKING

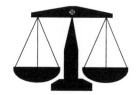

The BEST solution is one that:

✓ Solves the Problem

✓ Maximizes Positive Consequences

✓ Minimizes Negative Consequences

Evaluate Each Solution According to:

✓ Personal Consequences   ✓ Social Consequences

✓ Short-term Consequences   ✓ Long-term Consequences

✓ Likelihood that solution will solve the problem

✓ Likelihood that you can actually carry out solution optimally

Choose Solution with more pluses (+) than minuses (-)

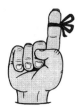

Decision-making tasks handout.

stuck in a dangerous place on the road, something bad could happen to the family if I walked for gas, we could make it to the movies and have a good time.

4. *What are the possible long-term effects?* I would learn my lesson to always have at least one-half tank of gas, we'd see the movie, but then no gas station would be open after the movie, the car engine could get damaged, the family would tease me for a long time.

It is not uncommon for some patients to automatically respond "I would never do it!" when told to evaluate the alternative "Do not stop!" Such patients are reminded that they will have their opportunity to evaluate the likelihood of implementing this option. However, they should first explore the possible consequences of such a solution because doing so may improve the ultimate solution plan decided on. Thinking about the positive and negative consequences of a variety of options may result in clarifying desired positive and negative consequences and actually lead to new ideas.

The therapist should assure the patient that, although the DM process initially seems time consuming, practice will facilitate the application of these steps in a more timely fashion. Initially, the slow-motion pace is necessary to illustrate the subtle benefits of coping with stressful problems in a more systematic and planful way. Not all decisions in the future will have to be made by using the worksheets provided. As the patient's skills become refined, he or she can decide when using a worksheet and recording the process is necessary. In our experience, patients choose to use the provided worksheets to increase their adherence to the systematic process when solving complex or particularly emotion-laden problems.

DEVELOPING AN OVERALL SOLUTION PLAN

Thus far, the patient has learned to identify, predict, and evaluate consequences that may result from implementing various alternatives. Each alternative is then evaluated for the likelihood that it would meet the patient's goals and whether he or she could optimally implement such a solution. The final step in the DM component of problem solving consists of bringing all of the previously mentioned strategies together in an effort to develop an overall solution plan. An optimal solution plan would also consist of the following: (a) combining alternatives or ideas to address various parts of the problem, and (b) devising a backup or contingency plan to rely on if the initial strategies do not meet the desired goals.

In developing an overall solution plan, the therapist directs the patient to choose those alternatives that best meet the criteria for effective problem resolution. Reiterating the definition for an effective solution (i.e., one that solves the problem, maximizes positive consequences, and minimizes negative consequences), the therapist assists the patient in reviewing the DM worksheet. The cost–benefit analysis, thus far, has considered each alternative independent of the others. The selection of an overall solution plan requires an objective comparison of the solution options on the basis of the positive and negative consequences predicted. Alternatives that were predicted to be "very unlikely" to meet the defined problem-solving goal are likely to be eliminated immediately.

For the remaining options, the number of pluses and minuses designated for each alternative are tallied across factors (i.e., personal, social, and short- and long-term consequences) on the DM worksheet. A potentially effective alternative would be represented by those ideas characterized by more pluses than minuses. Such ideas are considered to possess the greatest utility and serve as the basis of a potential solution plan to be implemented. The patient should be encouraged to select a combination of potentially effective solution options for the following reasons. First, there may be more than one alternative that is characterized by many pluses and few minuses. Thus, even if there is clearly one alternative with more pluses, complementing this solution with positive factors from another may enhance the efficacy of the overall solution plan. Second, it is likely that even an alternative predicted to result in many positive consequences may have areas of weakness. The patient can review the other alternatives to brainstorm new ways to overcome these weaknesses or to incorporate components of other alternatives into the most highly rated solution.

If it is unlikely that the patient could optimally carry out a solution (low likelihood estimate) that otherwise appears to have many positive consequences, the therapist and patient may reevaluate the obstacles preventing implementation. In such cases, subgoals may be developed to lead to the eventual implementation of this alternative if the obstacles could be overcome. For example, if a person with cancer would best have his or her needs met by a home nursing aide, but finances prevent hiring a private assistant, the use of the problem-solving process may be appropriate to meet the subgoal of "arranging finances to pay for an aide."

As mentioned throughout, the majority of complex real-life problems are likely to be composed of many factors that make it stressful or difficult. Therefore, an effective solution plan would be one that entails combining several alternatives, some of which address differing factors. In that manner, it is more likely that the problem will be solved completely and that the overall benefit picture becomes more positive. The solution plan should also specify when to carry out these various alternatives, either simultaneously or sequentially. If sequentially, which alternative is implemented first? Which one next? To make the most effective decision regarding the best method of carrying out an overall plan, we again recommend conducting a cost–benefit analysis of the various approaches.

Last, an effective plan provides for various contingency plans; that is, "If Plan A doesn't work, then do Plan B." In that manner, it is more likely that the problem will ultimately be solved, even if one's initial attempts are not successful.

What If No Alternatives Seem Likely to Work?

Patients should be prepared to expect that at times, their problem-solving efforts may not result in ideal or even acceptable solution plans on the first try. Although common sense may lead some individuals to this expectation, others will be discouraged, self-critical, or angry if they have not been forewarned of this possibility. Therefore, it is in the patients' best interest for therapists to discuss contingency planning proactively. In addition to better preparing patients, discussing the likelihood of occasionally experiencing unsuccessful problem-solving attempts helps to normalize the experience for them as well.

After reviewing the alternative solution options and conducting the cost–benefit analysis, there will be times when even the best combination of ideas does not meet the criteria for an effective solution plan. In such cases, patients are encouraged to reevaluate each component of their problem-solving process. Although the therapist has likely reminded them of the recursive nature of problem solving, the opportunity presents itself again. Patients should be prompted to recall the idea that problem solving often involves going back and forth among the different steps before problems are actually solved. For example, it is possible that the problem originally identified may need to be clarified or redefined altogether. Or, perhaps the goals stated at the outset of problem solving have changed or need to be broken down into more realistic, obtainable subgoals. If the definition remains unchanged and the goals seem appropriate on reevaluation, patients may attempt to generate more alternatives, either by brainstorming alone or by gathering new ideas from others.

Some clients may use problem-solving "failures" to validate their own cognitive distortions or irrational self-statements (i.e., "I knew I would be no good at this," "I'll never be able to cope better," or "This situation really is hopeless"). Having already invested a substantial amount of time in the process, patients should be reminded that reevaluating their previous efforts will lead them to make more rational and systematic decisions regarding their ability to solve this problem on their own. If the problem definition cannot be refined, the goals appear to be realistic, and every brainstorming strategy and tactic has been explored, the option of seeking professional help remains.

Seeking professional help after problem-solving efforts have not produced sufficient resolutions to problems can be viewed as another learning opportunity, rather than proof of failure. Patients are encouraged to be active in the process of receiving professional aid in solving their problems. Rather than allowing their problem to be solved for them, patients can request professionals to demonstrate or discuss the steps that they will take to lead them to problem resolution. For example, physicians are often willing to describe the procedures that they will perform during surgery or radiation in as much detail as patients are able to understand. Computer experts may explain the quirks of certain programs that they have learned to overcome through specialty training and experience. Similarly, accountants review tax forms and budgets with clients after they have completed their service. In some cases, patients may be able to perform the steps taken by the professional in the future if the opportunity presents itself again (i.e., self-care/maintenance of an infusion port). In other cases, professional assistance may always be required in response to a particular problem (i.e., high fevers). Regardless, patients may still advance their own knowledge about a particular problem and its resolution. Even when they are unable to resolve certain problems, they will at least have a rational understanding of why they were incapable of doing so.

Clinical Case: Gary

As Gary had described during his initial interview, he and his wife had significant financial concerns that would increase during his hospitalization. In addition to the fear of not being able to have money to pay utility bills, mortgage payments, and living expenses, Gary also described feelings of insecurity. He explained how his role in his marital relationship was being threatened by his inability to work. If his wife were to accompany him during his out-of-town hospitalization for the transplant, she would also be unable to work. Gary concentrated on this problem as a homework assignment after learning the DM skills. He completed PDF, GOA, and DM worksheets. He also drafted a list to separate his irrational thoughts or assumptions from the facts pertaining to this problem that helped him to organize his feelings of insecurity as a separate problem from the financial concerns.

Gary's approach to completing the DM worksheet demonstrates a useful variation of that exemplified previously. He defined the problem as "Celia and I only have my disability money to pay for our expenses if neither of us is working. This is a problem because we have payments to make in addition to the copayments and bills for my medical care that are adding up." Gary's goal was stated clearly in realistic and objective terms. He aimed to "generate enough income while he was in the hospital and recovering to be sure that he and his wife could cover their essential expenses (e.g., mortgage, food, and utilities) until they could both go back to work." Obstacles included (a) his inability to be in the public domain for approximately 6 months while his immunity is low and he is recovering from transplant; (b) Celia's inability to work if she stays with him in the hospital; (c) poor credit history, which prevented them from taking loans or a second mortgage; and (d) absence of family members who would be able to help them during this time.

Gary explained how writing more detailed information helped him to clarify his thoughts with regard to predicting consequences. He found that he needed to follow the strategies for DM in a step-by-step fashion to prevent himself from getting overwhelmed or impulsively skipping important components of the process. Therefore, Gary organized his work on two worksheets. On the first worksheet (see Exhibit 8.1), Gary listed the details of the consequences he predicted for each alternative solution. Next, he reviewed this list and used a highlighter to draw attention to the positive consequences that could result from implementing each solution (illustrated in italic text). By underscoring the positive consequences, he was able to evaluate his overall list to look for attributes that he would like to strive for in choosing his overall DM plan. Finally, Gary used the DM worksheet given by his therapist to conduct his cost–benefit analysis of the alternatives he was evaluating (see Figure 8.4). The following discussion ensued after the therapist looked over Gary's written work.

THERAPIST.   Gary, it seems like you've spent a lot of time thinking about your options, and I'm glad you wrote everything down so that we can talk about it today. This is very different from the way you described your attempts to solve problems in the past. How did this feel for you?

GARY.   When I work on the sheets like this I feel like I'm at least doing something about my problems. And that feels good.

THERAPIST.   You seem to put a lot of effort into learning these skills and the work we're doing in here. I'm really glad to see that.

GARY.   Well, right now I have time on my hands before I go to the hospital. A lot's on my mind and I'm trying to take care of some things. I have so many problems to think about that I want to do things right so I don't make everything worse.

EXHIBIT 8.1

Gary's Decision-Making Worksheet

"How can I generate enough income while in the hospital and recovering to be sure that my wife and I could cover our essential expenses (mortgage, food, and utilities) until we could both go back to work?"

▪ Take an advance on paychecks from work
Personal effects
I wouldn't feel good about this because when I go back to work I'd need money then too and I wouldn't be able to catch up.
Social effects
Celia would be worried about more debt. If I don't make it through this treatment, then she is stuck without money and with owing my boss. Also, my boss would probably expect me back to work sooner.
Short term effects
I would have money. I would be stressed about how I got the money.
Long-term effects
Hard to tell because I don't know how I'll be after treatment. But probably the long-term effects wouldn't be good because I'd have more debt again.

▪ Have Celia keep working and not come to hospital during my treatment
Personal effects
I would be very depressed and alone. Scared. Feel bad that she has to work and I can't.
Social effects
Celia would be okay with working, but not okay with not being with me. She would worry more. Person who is supposed to fill in for her while she is gone would have to find another job if she doesn't take off.
Short-term effects
Celia would be torn in different directions. *Could pay most of our bills.* Phone bills would be bigger because calls would be long distance for us to talk to each other.
Long-term effects
If I don't make it through the treatment, Celia will not forgive herself for not being with me. She will feel guilty. *Will have less debt. Celia may be able to take a break from working when I get out of the hospital, then she could be with me,* and I could try to work for awhile.

▪ Talk to social worker about money problems
Personal effects
Would feel good about having someone to help. Maybe I would be less anxious.
Social effects
Celia may feel better if we talk to someone else. No effect either way on social worker because it's his job, maybe he'd feel good about helping. *Wouldn't have to rely on boss or on Celia's workplace* (few negatives on others).
Short-term effects
May get some help. Maybe he has ideas that will help us get money, or could help to put off our bills. I'd feel like I'm doing something about the problem. Could reduce both Celia's and my worries about this. Would have more information.
Long-term effects
Maybe some of the cancer organizations give money so then we wouldn't have to pay it back *(less debt).* Make me more likely to help others if I get through this.

Continued

EXHIBIT 8.1 *Continued*

■ Have my sponsor get some AA members or neighborhood or coworkers together to help raise money for me. (Could have bake sale, sell coupon books, have a fund-raiser baseball game, collect door to door.)
Personal effects
 Afraid no one would do it. *Would feel good if people would do something like that for me*, but would feel bad that they'd have to do so much work. I would be kind of embarrassed for everyone to know that I'm broke.
Social effects
 Might put people out if they have to give up their money. Other people have money problems too. People might feel bad if they can't give money or *feel good if they do*. It would be a lot of work for my sponsor, but it was his idea. *Celia could help with the fundraiser and that would make her feel like she was able to do something for me.*
Short-term effects
 It would take a lot of time to organize something like that. It may take a lot of time to raise the money and the bills would be unpaid in the meantime. I would still feel like I wasn't doing anything about my own problem. *Wouldn't have to pay taxes on the money because it would be a gift.*
Long-term effects
 I might make some new friends. Celia would have more support both while I'm sick and if I don't get better. The money would definitely help!

THERAPIST. I think that's a good attitude to have—trying to prevent more problems and taking care of things the best that you can so that your stress eases up before you go in for your treatment. Let's talk about the work that you've done on your specific financial problem. You filled out the worksheet and did a lot of writing about the predicted consequences. After you did all of this, what did you come up with for your "solution plan?"

GARY. That's kind of where I got stuck. Most of the options had some good points about them. Like talking to the social worker, that seems like it would be good, and I could do it, but I'm not sure what the outcome really would be. Or the one about the fund-raiser. I think it would be really helpful if it worked out. My sponsor offered to set one up once. We didn't really talk about it at the time though, so I don't know how serious he is about it. I also don't know how other people would feel about it, I can see both kinds of reactions from it.

THERAPIST. Okay. Good, I'm glad these questions are coming up because they're important. Let's take them one at a time, starting with talking to your social worker. You know for a fact

FIGURE 8.4

DECISION-MAKING WORKSHEET

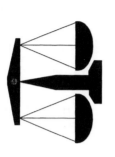

Instructions: (1) Write the problem-solving goal
(2) Write an abbreviated form of each alternative
(3) Predict and identify consequences of implementing each alternative
(4) Evaluate each alternative using the following rating scale

Rating Scale: + = *generally positive consequences; very likely*
– = *generally negative consequences; not very likely;*
0 = *neutral*

Goal: How can I ...   *Make money to cover expenses while in the hospital*

Alternative	Personal Effects	Social Effects	Short-term Effects	Long-term Effects	Likelihood of Success (Will it work?)	Likelihood of Implementation (Can I do it?)
Take an advance on paychecks from work					*in short term*	
Have Celia keep working and not come to the hospital during my treatment (6 weeks)						
Talk to the social worker about money problems						
Have sponsor and/or others have a fund-raiser		*Hard to decide for others*	*Not sure*			

Gary's completed decision-making worksheet.

that you have a social worker available to you, but you don't know what resources are available for him to offer you, right?

GARY.   Right.

THERAPIST.   So for now you're not really sure about the impact your conversation with Mark [the social worker] will have on your problem of needing money to pay your bills.

GARY.   Well, I guess that's true. I don't know if that will solve the problem, but it might.

THERAPIST.   You're right, it may solve the problem or it may not. The question to ask yourself is, "What are the positive and negative consequences of talking to Mark?" This will help you determine whether or not it is worth talking to him. Judging by what you've said already—you've met him, he seems nice, he mentioned something about finances—it sounds like talking to him wouldn't cause any negative consequences. Does that sound right?

GARY.   Yeah. I get that part. I guess where I got stuck is not wanting to choose that option because if it doesn't work I'm back at square one again.

THERAPIST.   What I think I hear you saying is that you don't want to put all of your eggs in one basket when you're not certain of the outcome?

GARY.   Exactly.

THERAPIST.   Is there any reason you could only choose that option?

GARY.   I don't think so. Except that I was afraid if I chose too many of these I would be taking on too much again, and that could be too stressful.

THERAPIST.   You're absolutely right about having to be aware of your own limitations. So let's evaluate what would happen if you combined several of these ideas. Which ones were you thinking of?

GARY.   Talking to the social worker and talking to my boss about working at home. Those two I could probably handle in terms of time. I mean it's really just two appointments. But then with the fund-raiser I got stuck because I guess I wasn't sure how to evaluate the social effects or the short-term effects.

THERAPIST.   What made it difficult for you?

GARY.   Well, I felt like I was just guessing and I didn't really have anything to base my pluses and minuses on.

THERAPIST.   Take it a bit further. Why do you think you felt that way?

GARY.   Because I don't really know how willing these people would be to do this for me.

THERAPIST.   And what's the best way to find out?

GARY.   [Smiles.] Ask them. I guess I need to get more information there!

THERAPIST.   You answered your own question very nicely! When you do get that information you will be able to make your decision easier. The important thing I want to point out here is to remember that combining ideas is actually one of the strategies to make your overall solution plan the best it can be. Of course you don't want to overwhelm yourself, but you also don't have to do everything at once, right? We can spend some time talking about prioritizing your alternatives. Before we do that, can you recall what we talked about when we talked about the optimal solution plan?

GARY.   Yeah. I have it written down. It's one that has the most pluses or positives, the least negatives, and gets at the problem from all sides. Thinking about the options I have, it really makes sense to try out a couple of these.

Clinical Commentary

Gary displayed his ability to follow the steps in the DM process. He tended to take information quite literally or concretely. Therefore, the therapist needed to lead him through the thought process about combining ideas to make a more effective overall plan and about recognizing the limits to his information. Most of all, Gary had little self-confidence about his DM ability because of the many failures in his past. Validating the work that he had done and reinforcing his ability to problem solve the difficulties that arose during the homework were key themes revisited throughout his therapy. Gary and the therapist spent an additional session talking about prioritizing goals and focusing his efforts. In the session, the therapist identified Gary's fear of failing at his attempts to use the problem-solving strategies. He agreed with this, as he believed he had no other coping mechanisms other than returning to alcohol use. The therapist guided him through the process of challenging these thoughts and combating them with positive statements. Furthermore, the therapist assured Gary that they would spend more time on this topic when they discussed solution implementation and verification.

PRACTICE WITH PERSONALLY RELEVANT PROBLEMS

The importance of practicing with personally relevant problems cannot be overemphasized. Allotment of time during training to apply the DM skills to personally relevant problems, in addition to the recommended practice exercise(s), is imperative to the patient's learning. However, the therapist should limit the initial problems addressed to those that can be completed within the introductory session(s). Problems that are too complex or that require extensive time dedicated to PDF or GOA should be saved for homework or a later session.

At first, the therapist acts as a team member during the initial practice attempts. As the patient's skills increase, the therapist will be required to do less modeling of the DM strategies and will assume the role of a coach. It is likely, even after in-session practice, that the patient will encounter new difficulties when he or she first attempts to apply the DM skills on his or her own. Therefore, the therapist should expect to allot time for practice of personally relevant problems in subsequent therapy sessions as well.

Clinical Trouble-shooting

The following are some difficulties that we have encountered during DM training, along with possible therapeutic responses.

- *Patient has difficulty believing immediate or "gut" reactions are less effective.* To illustrate a strategy to respond to this problem, consider John, a patient who exhibited an impulsive coping style and refuted this statement by claiming, "He who hesitates misses out!" John claimed that in dangerous or threatening situations, one's initial reaction may be what saves his life. He questioned the reality of being able to "hesitate" or contemplate one's actions in such situations. In this case, the therapist concurred that in extreme situations a modified or "emergency" problem-solving approach may be necessary. Yet, impulsive, "heroic" attempts often intensify or worsen such extreme situations. The therapist recognized John's tendency to be argumentative and skeptical. Before addressing this therapeutic phenomenon, the therapist encouraged John to provide an example from his own experience in which he thought his rationale applied. John described a confrontational situation

Clinical Trouble-shooting

continued

in which he raised his voice to his physical therapist, who suggested that he no longer needed physical therapy, that a gym membership would suffice. The patient could not afford such a luxury and therefore "caused a scene" in the physical therapist's office. Ultimately, the physical therapist agreed to allow him continued use of her facilities as a means of quieting him. John suggested that his approach to resolving this problem resulted in attainment of his goal (i.e., continued physical therapy). However, when the problem-solving therapist inquired about other resulting consequences, John admitted to being embarrassed by his actions and regretted the ill-feelings felt by his physical therapist and referring physician. Thus, in an overall reevaluation of his solution, he recognized the negative consequences that possibly could have been avoided if he engaged in the STOP and THINK strategy and considered another alternative solution.

▪ *Patient consistently evaluates all options negatively or with a neutral value.*

The therapist should address such a patient's ambivalence about solution options to identify the barrier to a realistic evaluation. Perhaps the problem is not significant to the patient. Furthermore, if a situation was a problem earlier in treatment, but resolved shortly after, and the therapist continues to revert back to this situation for practice exercises in future sessions, the patient may lose interest in applying the skills to this resolved situation.

In addition, options that are consistently rated with neutral values may indicate that the patient does not have clear expectations or goals for problem resolution. Therefore, the patient may be basing choices on nonaversive options or lack of negative consequences, rather than striving for positive results. A patient who consistently evaluates options from an unrealistically positive orientation may be avoiding thoughts about potential negative consequences. Or, perhaps more information is necessary to evaluate the situation at hand accurately. A patient who consistently evaluates options to all problems negatively may benefit from more concentrated sessions on problem orientation aspects, if DM appears to be biased.

Summary

We began this chapter with two quotations to emphasize the importance of reflective and consequential thinking. At the risk of going overboard, but because of its major importance, we add two more quotes to this list to continue to underscore the need to engage in the types of DM tasks outlined in this chapter:

> "Logical consequences are the scarecrows of fools and the beacons of wise men" (Thomas Henry Huxley, a nineteenth-century biologist) and "A thought which does not result in an action is nothing much, and an action which does not proceed from a thought is nothing at all" (Georges Bernanos, the twentieth-century French novelist we cited earlier in chapter 6).

Key Training Points

- Teach patient to identify the wide range of consequences (personal, social, short term, and long term) of each given alternative idea
- Help patient to make estimates of the value and likelihood of these various consequences
- Use "easier" problems initially as practice examples
- Teach patient to develop an overall solution plan that addresses multiple factors associated with a problem
- Emphasize notion that solution plan should contain backup plans
- Practice DM tasks with personally relevant problems

Suggested Handouts

- List of DM strategies
- DM worksheet

Homework

- By this point in the therapeutic process, patients expect new homework assignments to follow each session. Therapists should personalize these assignments to the extent necessary to help patients overcome difficulties in problem solving or specific to topics discussed in session. For example, if a patient recognizes the need for additional information to evaluate alternative solutions, he or she should be instructed to gather this information prior to the next training session.
- With regard to homework assignments at this juncture of training, we have asked patients to apply the problem-solving skills to two new problems that arise during the upcoming time until the next session. This assignment requires the completion of two of each of the following worksheets: PDF, GOA, and DM. The impor-

tance of practice should routinely be emphasized. Thus, if patients wish to complete additional worksheets, their diligent efforts and commitment should be reinforced.

Group Tips

- Practice of DM in a group of people with related experiences provides the unique opportunity for members to gain more information about predicted consequences from others who may have had to make similar decisions in the past. The group facilitator, however, should help members to keep experiences in perspective by evaluating the idiosyncratic nature of the information provided. Thus, practice exercises in a group can help people recognize the individuality of DM, reinforce the importance of separating factual information from assumptions, and consider the source of available information.

- Instruct participants to adopt investigative roles when helping others practice DM skills instead of predicting consequences to each other's solution options. For example, if a group member states, "Your family will get angry if you do that!" the therapist should facilitate participants' inquiry of their predictions, "How will your family react to that decision?" The inquisitor will gain practice in gathering information, rather than assuming particular outcomes, and the problem solver will have an opportunity for reflective thinking.

- Remind group members that they will likely differ in their assignment of value estimates because of individual differences.

Solution Implementation and Verification | 9

Overview

S olution implementation and verification (SIV) represents the fourth and last of the rational problem-solving skills. SIV training teaches patients to (a) optimally carry out a solution plan, (b) monitor the consequences of this implemented solution, (c) evaluate the actual outcome, (d) engage in self-reinforcement if the problem is solved, and (e) troubleshoot if the outcome is unsatisfactory. Introducing these skills concludes the presentation of new information with regard to problem solving. However, the cyclical and recursive nature of problem solving may lead the problem solver to revisit several or all of the previous components of the process in attempting to resolve specific problems. Problem orientation variables are discussed during SIV training specific to the hesitancy many people experience prior to implementing a solution, as well as issues of approach–avoidance.

Presenting the Rationale

As in previous training, to introduce the theory behind the SIV component of problem solving, we suggest the use of examples or slogans. A quote and an analogy that we have found to convey successfully the purpose of this training are provided, respectively, in the following paragraph.

> "The proof of the pudding is in the eating" (Miguel de Cervantes, the sixteenth-century Spanish novelist) and "One can study the game of tennis, practice swinging, and hit many balls against a wall, but until he faces his opponent on the court, he cannot win the game."

The following rationale may provide a useful example for therapists to paraphrase when explaining the SIV component to patients.

> So far in training, you learned to adopt a more positive approach to problem solving, better define problems, generate a comprehensive list of alternative solutions, and conduct a cost–benefit analysis of these options in order to make better decisions about which ideas to select as the best overall solution plan. Now is the time to begin carrying out the solution! As the ancient Chinese proverb states, "Be resolved and the thing is done!" In addition, I am suggesting that it is important not only to carry out the solution plan, but also to monitor and evaluate its effects.

> When making decisions, you also made predictions about the consequences or impact of the solution. Many people, when solving problems, often simply carry out the solution and hope for the best. However, by evaluating the consequences, we can better pinpoint where we went wrong if the solution isn't working. For example, if you decide to change your spending habits as one means of increasing your savings, you would keep financial records to determine if your plan is working. People trying to lose weight would weigh themselves to see if a diet is working. Doctors will monitor your symptoms to see if the cancer treatment is working. On the basis of the actual results, you might consider the problem solved or need to determine what went wrong if the problem is not solved.

The therapist should preface the following training exercises with a brief outline of the activities that make up this problem-solving task. Namely, the goals of this training component is for the patient to (a) learn how to carry out a solution plan optimally, (b) observe and monitor the actual outcome, (c) evaluate these results, and (d) self-reinforce or troubleshoot as necessary. A handout listing these components of SIV is contained in Figure 9.1.

Training in Solution Implementation

The problem-solving efforts extended thus far are worthwhile only if the solution plan comes to fruition. If a solution plan remains idle,

FIGURE 9.1

SOLUTION IMPLEMENTATION AND VERIFICATION TASKS

Carry out the Solution

 Observe and Monitor the Results

Evaluate the Results

Reward

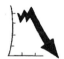 versus Troubleshoot

Get Professional Help

Solution implementation and verification tasks handout.

then the problem continues to exist or gets worse (i.e., the downward spiral of negative events). Therefore, carrying out the solution plan is a significant step to overcoming problems. Most people recognize the natural progression of this problem-solving process in theory. However, certain negative problem orientation factors may interfere with one's perceived ability to implement the solution plan that was developed. Examples of barriers to implementation may include fear of rejection, fear of success or failure, low self-efficacy, anxiety, denial, or avoidance.

To prepare patients to overcome self-imposed obstacles to implementing solutions, the therapist should discuss such factors during this training segment. Patients may or may not identify solution implementation as a problem for themselves; however, the following strategy can be beneficial to most people. If a person does not exhibit an avoidant coping style, the exercise can be viewed as a motivational strategy to carry out the solution plan optimally and in a timely manner.

SOLUTION IMPLEMENTATION TRAINING EXERCISE

During the DM process, patients are encouraged to evaluate the importance of resolving each particular problem at hand. This is also encouraged during SIV training, but in a less detailed manner as that conducted during the cost–benefit analysis. The Solution Implementation Worksheet, as shown in Figure 9.2, should be used to record the product of this exercise.

Patients are first instructed to brainstorm a list of consequences that are likely to result if the problem is not solved. Given that the problem was enough of a priority for patients to engage in problem-solving activities, it is likely that the list of predicted consequences of not solving the problem will resemble the patients' initial complaints. For example, Matt, an 18-year-old male cancer patient who was having extreme difficulty in making treatment decisions, replied to this prompt by stating, "Well, if I don't make this decision, then the cancer will make the decision for me, and I will no longer have a choice about what happens to me!"

Going beyond the limits of their presenting problems, patients are instructed to brainstorm a comprehensive list of other realistic consequences that are likely to result from not resolving the problem. During this task, patients are reminded to use their brainstorming skills and to focus also on the skills that they have learned during DM

FIGURE 9.2

SOLUTION IMPLEMENTATION WORKSHEET

Procrastination is the thief of time

Instructions. In Column A, list as many possible outcomes that you can identify that might occur if your problem is *not* solved. In Column B, list those positive effects that may occur if the problem is resolved. You may wish to use the ***brainstorming principles*** to help make these lists. Next, compare these consequences in order to answer the question– *Should I really avoid trying to solve this problem?*

A. Consequences if problem is *not* solved	B. Predicted consequences of chosen solution plan

Solution implementation worksheet handout.

training. Specifically, patients should brainstorm the likely personal, social, and short- and long-term consequences of not solving the problem. During SIV training, the therapist aids patients in monitoring this final list to ensure that the predicted consequences represent realistic effects of not solving the problem, rather than a list of unrealistic, negatively biased consequences. It is important for patients to learn to recognize this difference when engaging in this solution implementation exercise. Otherwise, patients with a tendency to evaluate problems and solutions negatively will provide themselves with false evidence that their problems are hopeless or that they are incapable of overcoming them. On the contrary, the purpose of this list of predicted outcomes is to highlight and remind patients of the risks and costs involved in not solving the problem, in comparison to the benefits and relief that they will experience if they do solve the problem. Thus, the next step in this exercise is for patients to list and review the predicted consequences that will result from solving their identified difficulties.

In developing the list of predicted consequences likely to result from problem resolution, patients may again use the visualization exercise taught earlier to imagine how life would be different for them and those involved, if their problem is resolved. In addition, patients can refer to their cost–benefit analysis drafted earlier for the particular solution plan they have selected.

This exercise should produce self-generated lists of reasons why particular problems should be resolved in a timely manner. Furthermore, patients will have "tipped the scales" of their cost–benefit analysis in such a way that the entire list of predicted consequences (if the problem is or is not resolved) should support the identified need to carry out the solution plan that they have already invested much time in creating. Patients often have more difficulty justifying procrastination or avoidance to themselves when they have constructed their own written evidence that solving their problem with the plan devised is in their best interest; to not do so would be deleterious.

If the solution plan requires an ongoing effort, rather than a point-in-time intervention, patients risk losing their motivation to follow through with their plan on a regular basis (e.g., complying with dietary restrictions, managing stress more effectively, or setting limits to prevent overcommitment). In such cases, therapists should brainstorm ideas with the patient to maximize the likelihood that he or she will benefit from this exercise. For example, we have encouraged patients to transcribe their lists of consequences onto 3 × 5 index cards and carry them in their wallet where they are continuously confronted with this information. Other individuals have posted their lists on bulletin boards to stimulate motivation. The following is a description of a 42-year-old female cancer patient, Gina, and is an example of how she benefited from this exercise.

Clinical Example: Gina

Gina had been working as an administrative assistant in a manufacturing company for 1 year prior to her diagnosis of breast cancer. She had a perfect attendance record, having never taken a sick day or reported late for work. After her diagnosis of cancer, Gina was determined not to allow her treatments to interfere with her responsibilities at work. She kept the details of her treatment and its effects private. The information Gina shared with her boss, Jana, was limited to treatment appointment schedules and her absenteeism following these dates. Although Gina felt that she was managing her responsibilities quite well, she recognized that her boss had begun to reduce her assignments. She no longer asked Gina to manage certain account files, and she had redirected the task of organizing upcoming client events to an account coordinator within the department.

Gina was upset and angry for her boss's failure to discuss these changes with her and for what she perceived as Jana's lack of faith in her ability to maintain her level of productivity during the course of cancer treatment. The first time she addressed this problem with Jana, Gina was reasonably satisfied that her boss would no longer overlook her willingness to accept new tasks. Jana had defended her actions by explaining that she was trying to be sympathetic to Gina's situation and permit her some flexibility to take time off as she needed. However, Gina used work as a distraction that enabled her to cope with her treatment and diagnosis and, therefore, did not want this designated "flexibility."

However, Jana continued to treat Gina differently, which led Gina to redefine her problem and her goals. As a result of her decision making, Gina decided that she needed to focus on her own perception of events as they occurred in the office. She identified her tendency to overanalyze her boss's behavior. Gina typically interpreted Jana's actions as personal attacks on her competence and commitment to her job and her overall well-being. She reacted adamantly against the stereotype of being "sickly" or weak. Gina also recognized that she needed to be more assertive when situations arose that made her upset or angry, particularly when her boss was contemplating the delegation of Gina's work to others. Gina's solution plan included focusing on her maladaptive appraisal of problems in her work environment and proactively addressing her boss when new activities came up for which she would like to be involved. This latter behavior would be in contrast to passively waiting to see who would receive a new assignment and then getting upset when the opportunity passed over her, which tended to be Gina's general reaction.

Clinical Dialogue

In the first session following DM, and prior to training in SIV, Gina described her frustration with her problem-solving efforts as follows:

GINA.   During the whole last week after we talked about my plan to deal with my boss and the work situation, nothing changed. I would go home at the end of the day and still get upset. But when these situations happened, I either didn't want to realize what was going on, or I totally chickened out of saying anything to my boss. Each day, I would tell myself things would get better, but they haven't. I guess part of it is I just can't get myself to face the problem when it's happening.

THERAPIST.   And you've reviewed your problem definition and your goal statement?

GINA.   Yes, and I think the problem is still there. My goals haven't changed any.

THERAPIST.   So, by not trying out your plan, you find yourself getting more frustrated and upset.

GINA.   Yes, I really do.

THERAPIST.   Actually, if you remember the end of our session last week, I briefly mentioned that we would be focusing on ways to help increase the likelihood that you would carry out the plan you've developed. Many people find themselves stuck in the same position that you find yourself in right now. It always seems easier to solve a problem in theory or on paper than it feels when you set out to solve the problem in real life. I think most people would agree with you. We are going to spend a good portion of the session today talking about the problems you've run into as far as getting started with your plan, and then talking about some skills that will help counter these obstacles. The exercises we do today should help you to overcome the difficulties you are experiencing with this problem, and those you encounter in the future.

The session proceeded, and the therapist began SIV skills training. Gina was particularly insightful about her hesitancy to address her problem. She was having difficulty overcoming her fear of getting her boss angry and her desire to be more assertive. Her lack of assertiveness had been a subgoal of her therapy and she had role-played various scenarios similar to the problems she was encountering at work. During the SIV training, Gina and her therapist focused on her avoidance of her present problem. After participating in the exercise of generating a list of consequences, Gina stated that she was more motivated to carry out her solution plan. When she returned the next week, she gave the following report:

GINA.   Well, I almost went through another week with the same problem that I've had this whole month. Monday night, I went home feeling very angry with myself for not speaking with my boss when I heard that the annual budget reports were due. I know they require a lot of time, but no one is more familiar with the paperwork than I am. If someone else does the report, it is likely that they will not use the system that I always do, and next year it will be a nightmare for me.

THERAPIST.   You said that you almost went through another week—did something change?

GINA.   Yes! I went home that night and read over the list we created last week. The one with all of the things that could happen if I continued to avoid the problem, and what could happen if I dealt with it. When I would read it, I felt like calling my boss at that moment. I would get ready to take action! The problem was I didn't feel like that when I was at work. So, what I decided to do was to take that list with me to work the next day. I put it in my top desk drawer where I keep pens, pencils, and notepads. That way I would see the list every time I opened the drawer. I really felt like I had a better attitude at work all day long.

THERAPIST.   That was a creative way to use the list to help you. And you say that your attitude improved?

GINA.   It did because it reminded me to STOP and THINK about what was going on and what would happen if I kept quiet about my feelings of being treated differently than I wanted to be. By Wednesday, I made an appointment with Jana! When we met later that day, she apologized to me for what's been going on. Now I really believe that she wasn't treating me differently on purpose. She told me that her sister-in-law had breast cancer before and she was trying to be sensitive to what she thought I must be going through. She gave me permission to be more vocal about what I think I can or cannot do.

THERAPIST.   How did you feel about the conversation with her this time?

GINA.   I tried to really listen to her and not be so focused on me. I can see that she means well. The funny thing is that she basically asked me to be more assertive!

THERAPIST.   I know this has been an ongoing struggle for you.

GINA.   It has, but I really think that if I keep looking at the list that I've made as a reminder of my goals, I have a better chance of trying to carry out some of the ideas that we've talked about.

THERAPIST.   You certainly sound more confident about what you need to do. Where will you go from here?

GINA.   The best I can say is that I'm really going to try to continue to carry out my plan—at least give it a chance.

Clinical Trouble-shooting

The following are difficulties that we have encountered in training and some possible therapeutic responses.

- *Patient perceives the risks of not carrying out the solution plan to be minimal in comparison to the effort necessary to change a situation.*

In some cases, a patient might complete a solution implementation worksheet and decide that few negative consequences would arise from doing nothing about a problem. If this should occur, the therapist and patient need to first review the list of consequences to ensure the validity of the patient's predictions. If the list of consequences appears realistic and comprehensive, other variables may need to be considered. In fact, the patient may have gained new information that negated the problematic nature of the situation as it first occurred. Alternatively, the therapist and patient may uncover other clinical issues. For example, in-depth discussion may reveal that the problem or goal the patient had chosen to focus on may have served as a distraction or attempt to avoid a larger problem. It is also possible that the patient has reconsidered the specific solution alternative chosen for implementation. During DM, the individual predicted and evaluated the consequences and likelihood of optimal implementation of each solution option. If at the time of implementation, the patient no longer believes that the assessment of the predicted consequences is accurate, the therapist may encourage the patient to select another alternative or to recycle through the various alternatives. However, recommendations should be suspended until the therapist and patient have had sufficient time to explore the nature of the change in motivation or desire to carry out a plan as previously outlined.

- *The patient's list of predicted consequences and benefits of carrying out the plan has not persuaded him or her to initiate implementation.*

  If a patient continues to be hesitant to carry out plans as self-designed, the therapist and patient should discuss perceived barriers to solution implementation. It is possible that some patients may have questions of their own competency to carry out specific solution plans; other patients may be doubting the efficacy of their own problem-solving ability and the likelihood that they could have generated a successful solution option.

GETTING READY TO CARRY OUT THE PLAN

On completion of the previous exercise, most patients should be in a position to implement the solution plan. Before initiating the problem-solving action, however, there are several suggested steps for patients to take to maximize the likelihood that the plan will be carried out optimally. Patients should be instructed to ask themselves, "What are the exact steps involved in the plan?" There are also several strategies that the therapist can use during this training or to present as examples to help patients evaluate the steps of their problem-solving plan on their own.

Strategy A

In session, the therapist may initially prompt patients by asking them to visualize a situation in which they initiate their problem-solving plan. Patients would then be asked to describe the scenario they envision to occur, beginning with their approach to the problem and continuing through its resolution.

Strategy B

If patients have difficulty with the visualization exercise, the therapist may supply open questions to model the thinking process that they should consider when they are functioning independently. These questions may be derived by use of the investigative reporter strategy, which was part of the earlier PDF training. For example, the therapist may ask several of the following questions: "*Who* do you need to speak with prior to implementing your plan?" "*What* tangible things do you need in order to implement your plan (e.g., date book to begin personal organization, grocery list to minimize purchases of frivolous or unhealthy foods, or suit from dry cleaners to wear for meeting with boss)?" "*Where* will you initiate the problem-solving attempt?" "*How* will you approach the situation?" "*What* happens when you are in the situation?" and "*What* do you do or not do?"

Strategy C

Patients may be asked to describe the details of their solution plan in a step-by-step fashion as if they were preparing a "user's manual" to solve a problem similar to their own. The audience of this manual is assumed to be people who are familiar with the problem situation, but who are unaware of the tactics and strategies that the patient chose to adopt.

Once the series of steps to implement the solution option have been decided on, patients are asked to consider any predicted or perceived obstacles that might have been uncovered during the previous exercise. Obstacles that might affect the problem solver's ability to carry out the solution plan in its optimal form should be evaluated. For example, a patient may have chosen to enroll in a yoga class for relaxation and stress reduction purposes. In considering the steps by which she would enroll and participate in the class, the patient learns that the class time conflicts with her husband's evening work shift. Therefore, the "transportation problem" needs to be resolved first, given that she is unable to drive herself and her husband is unavailable.

Patients may be given several guidelines by which to overcome newly identified obstacles to optimal solution implementation. Questions the therapist may ask include the following: "Are there ways to modify the solution plan which would overcome the obstacle (e.g., implement at a different time of the day, with different supports)?" and "Is there a direct approach by which the obstacle can be handled?" Depending on the magnitude of the obstacle and the severity of the impact it may have on the problem-solving attempt, patients may need to revisit previous problem-solving operations. The focus of the problem-solving efforts at this stage in the process may be to alter the existing plan, develop a new solution plan, or choose to temporarily postpone the implementation of a specific solution to develop a resolution to the identified obstacle or subgoal.

Practice or rehearsal of the hypothetical solution plan can improve patients' ability to reach the identified problem-solving goals with the least amount of difficulty. This principle is consistent with the message that the therapist should be reaffirming in each session; that is, asking patients to practice the problem-solving skills between sessions. Practice may take the form of going through the steps of the plan in the presence of a "neutral" person who can provide objective feedback. For example, a 27-year-old man, Bill, wanted to be discharged from the hospital into the care of his brother, Paul. Paul lived a long distance away from the hospital, and, therefore, frequent return visits to have his catheter lines flushed would be difficult to arrange. Reluctant to have home care nursing, Bill opted to learn to clean his ports and flush his lines on his own. To achieve his goal of semi-independence, Bill scheduled appointments with the home care team to practice flushing his lines under their supervision during the last week of his hospital admission.

Another form of practice is applying the steps of the solution plan to simulated tasks. This tactic is commonly used when patients are training to learn a new skill. For example, occupational therapists may help patients practice simulated tasks to improve upper body functioning. Simulations are also used to teach people to drive a car. If appropriate, patients can create their own simulated situations to practice the steps that they will carry out when the problematic situation occurs.

Role-play exercises and behavioral rehearsal are additional techniques to teach patients to help them prepare to carry out new problem-solving plans. Role-plays require the cooperation of another individual who is able to act as a *participant–observer*. For example, this individual would participate in the patient's practice attempts as a substitute for the person who will actually be involved in the solution (e.g., the subject of proposed conversation, individual who will directly be affected by the actions of the patient). The participant will also observe the patient's behavior or dialogue and provide feedback regarding the appropriateness of the patient's behavior and message. Rehearsal is a technique that is similar to role-play, but it does not necessarily require the presence of another. For example, many people use a mirror as an "audience" when rehearsing speeches or conversations.

Gina, the patient described previously, found role-play exercises particularly helpful to improve her confidence in confronting her boss, Jana, about her behavior. Gina asked a coworker of hers to anticipate Jana's response to her request for more responsibility. The coworker was able to provide Gina with a likely scenario that Gina may encounter. The opportunity for Gina to role-play several scenarios that might result from her conversation helped her to feel more prepared to be assertive and speak with her boss. She also benefited from the suggestions and feedback provided by her coworker.

SKILL DEFICITS RELATED TO SOLUTION PLAN

If skill deficits (i.e., problem-focused coping skills or emotion-focused coping skills) are identified and related to the designated solution plan, the strategies of solving the problem need to be reevaluated. Essentially, in keeping with the problem-solving model, the therapist is faced with deciding among the following options: (a) to incorporate the appropriate skills training into the therapy (or have it obtained outside of the therapy), (b) to instruct the patient to return to certain previous problem-solving operations (e.g., GOA and DM) to develop a new plan, or (c) to work with the patient to reformulate the overall definition of the problem situation to include the skill deficits as an obstacle to overcome in the overall solution plan of a particular identified problem. In essence, such a decision requires the therapist to engage in problem solving him- or herself with the overall goal of helping this particular patient with his or her given limitations and strengths to overcome the short-term problem identified, and the long-term goal of improving coping abilities in future problematic situations (see A. M. Nezu & Nezu, 1989, and C. M. Nezu & Nezu, 1995, for discussions of how a therapist can use the problem-solving principles to enhance clinical decision making). If the skill deficits identified are likely to interfere with future problem-solving efforts, the individual is likely to benefit from addressing these difficulties at some point in therapy.

Solution Verification

DEVELOPING A DATA COLLECTION SYSTEM

Monitoring the success of a solution plan maximizes the likelihood that the problem is resolved to patients' satisfaction or allows for subsequent modifications. This step in problem solving is often overlooked or ignored. Many people consider the implementation of a solution plan to be their last necessary effort. As mentioned earlier, patients often carry out their solution plan and simply hope for the best. It is also common to hear patients complain, "I did what I said I would, it didn't work, so I give up!" However, the therapist needs to convey that abandoning the problem-solving process after carrying out a solution plan is analogous to throwing the bowling ball down the lane and leaving the alley before it reaches the pins. Without evaluating the outcome of one's efforts, it is difficult to determine whether one's approach to solving a particular problem was successful or if additional work is necessary.

Monitoring the success of a solution plan requires the development of a *data collection system*. A data collection method should be simple, but comprehensive enough to measure the effects of the solution plan. Examples of commonly used data collection methods include keeping track of checking accounts to monitor expenditures and savings; using weight charts for dieting; calculating hitting averages for baseball players; and checking blood pressure, pulse rates, or tumor markers to monitor health status.

The problem-solving therapist provides the guidelines by which patients develop their own monitoring system. It is important that the actual techniques or methods to be used are derived by patients. The importance of this is twofold. First, patients are more likely to adhere to a plan, which is deemed reasonable and easy to remember, that they have devised themselves and to incorporate it into their lifestyle or schedule. Second, patients must be able to develop plans with some degree of autonomy if they are to generalize their problem-solving skills to future problems posttreatment.

The development of a monitoring system can be facilitated by using a combination of problem-solving skills. Patients are advised to use concrete, unambiguous language to outline their data collection system. The description of a data collection should describe the increments of change that they will measure (e.g., time, weight, money, commitments, obligations, phone calls, and pleasurable activities), the ultimate goal of the plan, and the actual consequences (i.e., personal, social, short term, and long term) of the implemented solution. Creativity, fostered by brainstorming principles, can enhance data collection systems by helping the person to think of personally appropriate methods.

Clinical Example: Jim

A tailored data collection system developed by a 34-year-old male cancer patient, Jim, involved monitoring the frequency of engaging in physical fitness activities as recommended by his oncologist. It was suggested that he increase his muscle strength and cardiovascular fitness to improve his ability to sustain extended periods of bed rest during the intervals of his chemotherapy treatments. Jim knew that he frequently viewed his monthly calender in his personal planner book. Therefore, he chose to use stickers of his favorite cartoon characters to mark the days in which he exercised so that he would routinely be greeted by a visual account of his plan in action. This monitoring system served to provide a quick reminder of his goal (i.e., to increase the frequency of gym use), reinforcement when he successfully met his goal of three stickers per week, and an easy way to track his efforts on a daily basis.

Clinical Commentary

Although Jim's plan accounted for the number of times he did or did not meet his goal, it only partially fulfilled the requirements for an optimal data collection system. His therapist addressed the importance of monitoring the consequences of solution plans, including the risks and benefits. Jim's plan was then complemented with a health chart on which he recorded his weight and blood pressure on a biweekly basis. In addition, he kept a log of his energy level by recording a score on a scale of 1 to 10 next to his cartoon sticker. The rationale for this addendum to his plan was to monitor the effects the exercise was having on his daily functioning. If he began to record more feelings of fatigue or less energy, he and his doctor could modify his workout regimen and redefine his exercise goals to develop a more appropriate fitness protocol. However, if Jim continued to monitor only the frequency of visits to the health club, he would have no qualitative or quantitative record of the change in his physical functioning.

SOLUTION VERIFICATION: EVALUATING THE RESULTS

Carefully documenting the resulting effects of solution plans allows for more effective evaluations of the overall success of problem-solving attempts. Specifically, the monitoring systems that patients develop should provide them with data to compare the *actual* consequences of their solution plans with the consequences that they *predicted* would occur during the DM process. The use of the solution verification worksheet (Figure 9.3) aids patients in this evaluation of their problem-solving outcomes.

By comparing the actual effects of implementing a solution plan with the predicted results, patients are led to the next step of the problem-solving process. Patients' self-evaluation of their attempts to solve problems may provide them with a sense of closure and resolution if the effects of the solution plan are favorable. Conversely, if the results of their solution plans do not match their predicted consequences or are not favorable, patients will be able to prepare themselves for troubleshooting.

GIVING SELF-REINFORCEMENT

If patients are successful in their problem-solving efforts, evaluating the actual resulting consequences allows them to acknowledge their accomplishment and helps them to accept responsibility for their productive and positive actions. To facilitate recognition of effective problem solving, the therapist should instruct patients to use self-reinforcement as an additional skill in the process of resolving problems. Self-reinforcement helps to underscore the importance of any and all problem-solving attempts. Planning a specific and desired form of self-

FIGURE 9.3

SOLUTION VERIFICATION WORKSHEET

A. What were the results of your solution plan?

B. How well did your solution meet your goals?

1	2	3	4	5
Not at all		Somewhat		Very Well

C. What were the actual effects on you (personal effects)?

D. How well did these effects match your original predictions about personal consequences?

1	2	3	4	5
Not at all		Somewhat		Very Well

E. What were the actual effects on others?

F. How well did these results match your original predictions about consequences concerning others?

1	2	3	4	5
Not at all		Somewhat		Very Well

OVERALL SATISFACTION WITH RESULTS

1	2	3	4	5
Not at all satisfied		Somewhat satisfied		Very Satisfied

Solution verification worksheet handout.

reinforcement as a reward for successfully overcoming a particular problem will also motivate patients to initiate problem-solving action in the future. Although the primary motivation for engaging in problem solving should be to reduce distress, overcome difficulties, and increase or decrease a particular behavior, feeling, or situation, self-reinforcement is intended to be a "bonus" for achieving goals.

Self-reinforcement can take many forms. A reinforcer may consist of a concrete reward such as purchasing a new object, engaging in a pleasurable activity, praising oneself, or relieving oneself of an obligation or chore. In our experience, patients have purchased record albums, clothes, sporting equipment, or computer products as rewards. Others have made time for themselves or allotted finances to engage in activities that they typically did not have the opportunity to enjoy (e.g., going to the movies, taking a day off from work, or sleeping later than usual). The temporary relief of certain obligations or stressors may also serve as a reward for some individuals. A 32-year-old mother, Anna, described her self-reinforcement as hiring a babysitter while she spent her day doing pleasurable activities for herself without the concern of her 4-year-old daughter. Patients should be encouraged to begin brainstorming a potential list of reinforcers while they are in session. As problem solving is initiated for different problems, the list of reinforcers may change to reflect a reward that is more closely related to overcoming the difficulty at hand (e.g., purchasing new clothes as the patient improves her body-image concerns after breast surgery).

The practice of self-reinforcement is particularly important for individuals who think of themselves as poor problem solvers and who have poor self-efficacy beliefs with regard to their ability to cope with difficult problems. Recognizing their ability to resolve a problem successfully will increase their belief that they will be able to handle difficult problems in the future. Furthermore, if patients increase their awareness of how the use of problem-solving skills aided them in reaching effective solutions, they will also be more likely to rely on these skills when other problems arise.

TROUBLESHOOTING WHEN PROBLEM-SOLVING EFFORTS ARE NOT SUCCESSFUL

Patients should be prepared during the training sessions to expect that everyone encounters situations in which their problems are not solved by the first solution plan attempted. The importance for the therapist to discuss this likelihood cannot be overstated. However, patients should also be reassured that after troubleshooting and recycling back through other problem-solving operations, most problems do get resolved. Therefore, having implemented a solution plan that results in less than optimal consequences is not a reason for giving up. Those whose solution plans were not found to be effective should follow the course of *troubleshooting*.

Troubleshooting for patients means reviewing each step of the problem-solving process to identify areas in which the complications surfaced. Specific to solution implementation, troubleshooting refers to identifying the areas in which the actual consequences do not match the predicted consequences and subsequently attempting to understand why the discrepancy occurred. Having completed the solution verification worksheet, patients will be able to determine in which areas changes are necessary. For example, did the solution plan fail to achieve the desired personal effects, social effects, or goal attainment? Evaluation of the difficulties that arose will lead to a quicker optimal resolution than immediately dismissing their entire problem-solving effort as a failure. By choosing not to review the problem-solving steps and overall solution plan, patients risk repeating ineffective methods for coping with their problems. If patients do need to find new approaches by which to solve their problems, it is recommended that the entire set of problem-solving worksheets be used to increase the systematization of renewed attempts.

At times, patients may diligently recycle through the problem-solving process several times and still be displeased with their options for resolving certain problems. In such cases, professional assistance may be necessary to overcome unremitting problems. As described in the DM training session, patients are reminded that everyone, at certain times, needs the help of experts, especially in complex, unique, or very stressful situations. The need for such help should be viewed as an opportunity to learn new techniques, approaches, or skills to approach similar problems in the future. A review of problem orientation principles can help patients reframe their perception of resorting to professional help if this option is viewed unfavorably. Conversely, although patients must learn to recognize the limits of their abilities or skills, they should also be encouraged to make a reasonable effort to solve problems independently, rather than turning to others after initial unsuccessful attempts at problem resolution.

Clinical Example: Marianne

Marianne was a 31-year-old single mother who had been diagnosed with ovarian cancer. She and her 3-year-old daughter, Dana, were living with Marianne's mother after she became sick. Because of the effects of her disease, surgery, and treatment, Marianne was unable to assume the same level of responsibility for her daughter as she did prior to her illness. Her mother took Dana to her play group two times per week in place of Marianne. In the evening, when Marianne became tired earlier than usual, her mother read Dana a bedtime story.

Dana began misbehaving more frequently by screaming, pushing other children in her play group, and disobeying Marianne. Expecting to see some change in Dana's behavior because of her illness, Marianne used her problem-solving skills to generate creative ways to spend quality time with Dana. Marianne also attempted to explain to Dana that she was sick. However, after several unsuccessful efforts to discipline or calm Dana down, Marianne decided that solving her daughter's behavioral problems was beyond her abilities. Marianne became so frustrated that she feared she would physically harm her child. Therefore, she contacted a psychologist at the community mental health center who specialized in child behavior problems.

Marianne told her problem-solving therapist that she had been feeling overwhelmed by her child's misbehavior. She also acknowledged feelings of sadness and rejection from her daughter and guilt for taking her daughter to the mental health center. Although Marianne knew she has become more irritable because of her exhaustion and sickness, she also believed that she thoroughly explored her options to resolve her problem on her own.

Initially, Marianne began to doubt her ability to apply her problem-solving skills to cope with serious problems. After discussing these feelings with her therapist, however, she was able to reframe her actions more positively. Marianne realized that not only did she initiate effective action by taking her daughter to the clinic but that she also minimized the opportunity for her to lose her temper with her daughter and cause more damage to their relationship.

Clinical Commentary

Dana was referred to another psychologist within the clinic who conducted support groups for children of patients with chronic illnesses. The psychologist explained to Marianne some of the common reactions expressed by children of Dana's age. In combination with suggestions for home-based behavior modification techniques, Marianne felt more in control of her daughter's behavior, her own frustrations, and her ability to overcome this problem effectively.

PRACTICE IN SIV SKILLS

Practice during this stage of training may begin by reviewing solution plans decided on previously during the DM sessions. The therapist's role is to help patients anticipate potential obstacles that may interfere with the optimal implementation of the outlined solution plans. If patients decide that rehearsal, role-playing, or practice is necessary to ensure optimal implementation of a solution plan, the therapy session may be the ideal time to engage in this preparation. Additional problem solving may be required as well, on the basis of the obstacles that surface on review of the solution plan.

Obviously, it is difficult, if not impossible, for patients to carry out solutions to most personal problems within the therapy session. However, practice is important to ensure patients' understanding of the concepts introduced during SIV training. Thus, the solution implementation worksheet should be completed on several problems that have continued to be the focus of the therapy or new problems that were detailed in the previous homework assignment(s). Some patients may be hesitant or reluctant to carry out their proposed solution plans for given problems. Regardless of confidence or motivation to implement specific solution plans, every patient should complete the SIV worksheet for the purpose of discussion and preparation for more challenging problems in the future.

Referring to the problems recently discussed in reviewing homework, patients and therapists can discuss the type of information that will be used to monitor the effects of implementing solution plans. Brainstorming ideas for data collection systems in session will also provide therapists with additional opportunities to evaluate patients' problem-solving skills. Therapists may aid patients in constructing data collection systems by supplying them with more examples if they initially have difficulty generating their own ideas. The bulk of the practice of SIV skills will occur outside of the session. Therefore, patients should be advised to keep copious notes of their attempts to implement and monitor solutions to be discussed in future sessions.

Clinical Case: Gary

In the session following SIV training, Gary reported the observed effects of two solution plans that he implemented. The first solution plan was in response to his financial problem as described in the DM session. The second plan was an attempt to discuss his marital problems with his wife. Both of these problems had been discussed in detail throughout Gary's problem-solving training. During SIV training, Gary acknowledged his anxiety about actually carrying out the solution plans he had constructed. In the previous session, the therapist assisted Gary in evaluating the thoughts that contributed to his fears of failure and rejection. A significant amount of time was also spent generating additional ideas and actions that would increase Gary's comfort level in implementing his solution plans.

Gary's Financial Problems

Gary had chosen to combine several ideas from his DM list to solve his financial problems that would arise during his hospitalization. He decided to monitor the outcome of his efforts to overcome his financial problems by keeping a log book. For each identified solution he intended to implement, Gary listed the anticipated or desired outcome. He then checked off each tactic he carried out. In keeping with the SIV worksheet, Gary rated the outcome of each action taken on a scale of 1 to 5. Several parts of his plan required follow-up phone calls or subsequent efforts, so he organized his solution plan charting record to accommodate the new list of activities likely to result.

Because of the complexity of his financial solution plan, Gary recognized the need for an inexpensive, simple, yet systematic way of tracking incoming money and bills paid out. He decided to purchase an accountant-style ledger book and asked a coworker for advice in organizing it. He requested his wife to be present when the accounting system was developed so she could accurately maintain it during his anticipated periods of debilitating illness. He reported this organization gave him a sense of accomplishment and decreased his anxiety about his wife temporarily handling their finances in the future.

Gary described the details of his efforts as follows. He spoke with his social worker who proved to be instrumental in negotiating payment plans for Gary's utility bills and cost of the transplant. The social worker also introduced Gary to the home-care coordinator to assess the anticipated medical needs and costs after his hospital discharge. Finally, the social worker provided Gary with new information regarding foundations and organizations that awarded monetary support to recipients of bone marrow transplants. Although these donations did not cover all of Gary's expenses, the money was not taxable and did not require repayment.

The second idea Gary pursued pertained to the fund-raisers. When Gary approached his AA sponsor, he was met with some reluctance. The sponsor wanted to help Gary raise money but did not have time to prepare or organize such an undertaking. However, the two men used brainstorming skills to overcome the time constriction. The conclusion of these discussions led Celia and Gary's sponsor to identify preestablished functions (e.g., community center sports leagues, bingo halls, and fast-food restaurants) where they could leave donation cans for people to deposit spare change. Ultimately, this option was quite profitable.

Last, Gary's boss was pleased to oblige Gary's desire to work from the hospital. His concern, however, was Gary's health and ability to concentrate on fine details. When Gary explained that his desire to work was based on need for distraction as well as financially driven, his boss was willing to offer Gary several options. Although the work that was given to Gary was not as challenging as he would have preferred, it allowed him to learn about a different facet of the company. His boss assured Gary that learning the basic procedures under this other division would enable him to advance quickly on his return.

Although two of Gary's options resulted in outcomes slightly different than he anticipated, the overall results of his problem-solving efforts to reduce his financial hardships were positive. Gary was realistic to expect that he would still accumulate many bills and have some debt as a result of his treatment and inability to work for an extended period of time. However, he substantially minimized the debt incurred during his disability. Most important, Gary was relieved of the worry that he would have to file bankruptcy or lose the mortgage on his house. He was confident that he would have "peace of mind" while in the hospital and that he could figure out a way to manage his finances and outstanding bills after his hospital stay.

Gary's Marital Problems

Next, Gary discussed the progress he had made in working on his marital problems. Specifically, he defined their problems as miscommunication or lack of communication at times, as well as a lack of intimacy. He explained that he and Celia had been cohabitating for the past few years as roommates rather than as spouses. Throughout Gary's diagnosis and treatment, however, he reevaluated their relationship. As Gary learned to better manage his anger, reduce his anxiety, and cope more effectively with problems, his mood also improved. Gary became thankful for the people in his life who helped him through his battle with cancer. Specifically, he valued Celia's devotion to him and willingness to support him during this difficult time. With these changes in feelings, Gary wondered whether their marriage could be revived. Yet, he feared approaching this topic with Celia because he did not know what type of reaction to anticipate.

After completing a set of problem-solving worksheets, Gary planned the optimal time to speak with Celia and carefully planned his words. He spent part of his therapy session role-playing his proposed dialogue with the therapist. To boost his confidence and motivate himself, Gary completed the solution implementation worksheet. His stated purpose for completing this particular worksheet (in addition to fulfilling his assignment) was "to prove to myself that I really had a lot more to gain than to lose." Recognizing that this conversation would surprise his wife, he made an "extra effort" to maintain realistic expectations for the outcome of their discussion.

Clinical Commentary

Gary presented his completed Solution Verification Worksheet to his therapist as contained in Figure 9.4. The results of Gary's discussion with his wife pleased him for two reasons. First, Gary was encouraged by his ability to follow through with his plan with much less anxiety than he typically experienced in uncertain situations. His self-efficacy improved and he became more hopeful that he could regain the quality of life he hoped for by using problem solving to overcome obstacles to achieving happiness. Second, his conversation with his wife served as a springboard to what he hoped would lead to reconciliation. In general, with much effort and perseverance, by using the various problem-solving principles and strategies, Gary began to successfully resolve major life problems, while simultaneously feeling better about his ability to do so.

Summary

The SIV process takes the patient from the theoretical to the applied. Patients are encouraged to begin to implement the chosen solution plan and to evaluate its effects. However, even though a contemporary sports ad contains a oft-cited piece of advice—"Just do it!—many people become reluctant to carry out their solution despite the amount of time and energy that had already gone into developing the solution plan. As such, inherent in SIV training is a motivational component and often may require the problem-solving therapist to recycle back to various problem orientation exercises to facilitate patients' willingness and resolve to implement the solution.

Moreover, carrying out the plan does not represent the final problem-solving step. Rather, patients are encouraged to monitor and evaluate the consequences of the solution. Depending on the outcome of this process, they are then encouraged to engage either in self-reinforcement (if the problem is solved) or in troubleshooting (if the problem is not resolved).

As in any skill, practice does makes perfect. Although we are far from advocating that patients become perfect at problem solving, we strongly advocate the notion of practice. Therefore, the remainder of the problem-solving sessions are devoted to practice, practice, practice, as described in the next chapter.

FIGURE 9.4

SOLUTION VERIFICATION WORKSHEET

A. What were the results of your solution plan?

Celia and I talked about our marriage for the first time in a long, long time. At first we argued a little about who was to blame for the way our marriage has been. I told her that I didn't want to fight, and then I just came out and told her what I wanted to say. She cried a little at first. We both agreed to talk about it more after she's had some time to think about what I said. We talked two days later. The result was that we still need to figure out how to get our marriage back on track, but we both want to try to work things out.

B. How well did your solution meet your goals?

1	2	3	4	5
Not at all		Somewhat		Very Well

C. What were the actual effects on you (personal effects)?

Before I talked to Celia I was really nervous and kind of scared. After we talked for the first time I was still kind of nervous because I wasn't sure exactly what she was thinking. But I felt really proud of myself for bringing it up to her. Actually, I wasn't even as nervous as I thought I would be. After we talked the second time, I cried a little too. For the first time in a long time I felt like we connected. I felt like I was taking charge of this problem. I was still nervous about what it might take to work things out, but overall I felt a lot better.

D. How well did these effects match your original predictions about personal consequences?

1	2	3	4	5
Not at all		Somewhat		Very Well

E. What were the actual effects on others?

Celia was shocked when I brought the conversation up to her. I think she didn't know what to think. I also think she was unsure if she should trust what I was saying, but I believe she wanted to. This was the first time that I initiated this conversation instead of her, so that pleased her. After our second talk I think she really knew I was sincere. The effect on her was good, but I also think she's a little guarded to get her hopes up that things will be really different.

F. How well did these results match your original predictions about consequences concerning others?

1	2	3	4	5
Not at all		Somewhat		Very Well

OVERALL SATISFACTION WITH RESULTS

1	2	3	4	5
Not at all satisfied		Somewhat satisfied		Very Satisfied

Gary's completed solution verification worksheet.

Key Training Points

- Facilitate patient's motivation to carry out solution plan using SIV worksheets
- If necessary, recycle back to various problem orientation exercises to help encourage patient to implement solution
- Have patient rehearse or role-play carrying out the solution when applicable to increase likelihood that he or she will optimally implement it in the future
- Help patient develop appropriate monitoring systems relevant to a particular problem and solution plan
- Teach patient to self-reinforce
- Teach patient to troubleshoot

Suggested Handouts

- SIV tasks
- Solution Implementation Worksheet
- Solution Verification Worksheet

Homework

- At the conclusion of the sessions devoted to SIV training, therapists should review the rationale and skills taught. Likewise, because of the reciprocal nature of the problem-solving process, it may be helpful for therapists to review the main points of each problem-solving component. Patients will have the opportunity to practice each of these skills for homework that will be due in the following session(s). Homework at the end of SIV training includes at least one entire set of rationale problem-solving skills worksheets (PDF, GOA, DM, and SIV) on a new problem. Thus, patients should identify a new problem that occurs and should attempt to solve the problem by using the systematic structure of the skills before the next session. As emphasized during each session, maintenance of a positive problem orientation is crucial to optimal completion of this homework assignment.

Group Tips

- Use group members to encourage one another when hesitant to carry out solution plans. Encourage them to help identify potential positive and negative consequences of not solving problems for each other.
- Engage group in multiple role-plays to have all group members practice carrying out solutions, especially if the plans involve any interpersonal aspects (e.g., talking to a spouse about a delicate subject). Group members should be encouraged to provide con

structive feedback to each other regarding a person's "performance." The group leader, however, should be the final judge of how the person performed.

- Have group members provide additional ideas about data collection systems for each other. This may involve a group brainstorming session, which could provide for additional practice in this skill.

- Group members can also engage in brainstorming to think of additional ideas for appropriate reinforcers.

Practice, Practice, Practice 10

Overview

After the major PST training has taken place, the remainder of treatment is devoted to practice. The importance of such practice is conveyed in the quote by thirteenth-century Persian poet Saadi, "However much thou art read in theory, if thou hast no practice, thou art ignorant." As with any new skill, the more one practices, the better one gets. Beyond actually solving stressful problems, continuous practice in this context serves three additional purposes: (a) Applying the problem-solving model under the "supervision" of a therapist allows for helpful professional feedback, (b) increased facility with the model through practice can decrease the amount of time and effort necessary to apply the entire model with each new problem, and (c) it helps to facilitate maintenance and generalization of the skills.

PRACTICE, PRACTICE, PRACTICE

The therapist's goals for these practice sessions are to (a) help the patients fine-tune the problem-solving skills that they have acquired, (b) monitor the patients' application of these principles, and (c) reinforce the patients' progress as a means of further increasing their sense of self-efficacy. The number of practice sessions required after formal training ends is dependent on the competency level that a patient achieves, as well as the actual improvement in his or her overall quality of life. According to our research protocol, we have allotted three additional sessions beyond specific training, but for open-ended situations, the problem-solving therapist can be more flexible with regard to changing this number. However, we do strongly encourage that some sessions devoted specifically to practice are included.

A typical practice session begins and ends in a similar manner as the previous skills-training sessions. Patients are asked to review how they applied the problem-solving skills to assigned or new problems since the past session, as well as to discuss areas that have been difficult for them. By this point, patients have been given several complete sets of problem-solving worksheets. If full sets have been completed, patients may be asked to self-evaluate strengths and difficulties in solving a given problem. Feedback should be provided as appropriate. If no further discussion is necessary regarding predicted negative consequences or prevention of similar problems in the future, then a new problem can be addressed. If, however, patients find that they could not complete the problem-solving worksheets because of confusion or feeling stuck, the remainder of the session should be spent identifying and addressing the obstacles encountered. Moreover, it is possible that the problem-solving therapist needs to return to certain ideas or training exercises previously introduced to enhance patients' understanding of a given issue or skill acquisition regarding a particular strategy.

The therapist is advised to continue evaluating and monitoring patients' motivation to practice the problem-solving skills. The importance of practice cannot be overemphasized. Yet, some patients may value practice sessions less than skills-training sessions because they misperceive the bulk of the necessary effort that is needed to be done. Other individuals may believe that the skills-training sessions adequately addressed the problems that brought them in for therapy and, therefore, no longer believe additional sessions are necessary. For these reasons, it is imperative that the purpose of the practice sessions be underscored at the end of SIV training. Patients should be encouraged to ask questions regarding the structure or content of these sessions. Furthermore, the therapist may wish to check in with the patients during these practice sessions to assess their perceived satisfaction and benefits resulting from the brief continuation of therapy. The structure and content of these sessions can be adjusted accordingly at the therapist's discretion.

Patients may choose to use these sessions to focus on aspects of problems that they had introduced earlier in their training that were not resolved or to address new problems for discussion. As a means of enhancing maintenance and generalization, potential problems that may occur in the future should also be discussed to help patients plan accordingly and to begin to associate the possibility of managing these difficulties by using the newly learned skills.

TERMINATION

When the therapist and the patient agree termination is appropriate, the therapist may wish to provide additional handouts for duplication and future use. During this final session, the therapist continues to process the closure of therapy and the therapeutic relationship. The therapist should review the initial goals of PST, as discussed in the first session. Patients may be asked for examples of how these goals have been met (e.g., "In what areas has the patient increased his or her sense of control?" and "Quality of life?"). Feedback regarding the therapist's perspective of treatment progress is also important. Areas of weaknesses and strengths may be addressed in review, and recommendations of how to maintain gains (i.e., practice or monitor self-improvement) should be made. Reinforcement is especially important in this final session, as patients often experience some trepidation about "losing" their support. Furthermore, patients often recall the most recent message given by the therapist and words of encouragement may be internalized as positive self-statements in future stressful situations. In general, patients should be encouraged to practice the problem-solving skills in as many day-to-day situations as possible to facilitate a true incorporation of the philosophy and skills underlying this approach into their daily thoughts, feelings, and actions.

PROBLEMS WITH TERMINATION

For some patients, termination itself may represent a "problem to be solved." In addressing these issues, therapeutic tactics for termination are built on the general strategy of helping patients to use learned problem-solving skills and to apply them to any problems concomitant with ending treatment. For example, problem orientation skills can be used when encountering feelings such as sadness, fear, anger, guilt, or relief. Such emotions are often mixed and represent a powerful signal to try to understand what is happening and that a problem exists. The use of skills involved in problem definition and formulation to acknowledge the loss of the therapy relationship and to define individual subproblems is an important next step toward resolving treatment termination difficulties. Each patient's goals for, and personal obstacles to, an optimal end of therapy can then be specified. After the goals and obstacles are clearly defined, various strategies can be generated to meet these goals. In this manner, the last session can serve as the time to self-monitor and evaluate the effectiveness of the strategies mutually chosen by the therapist and the patient to ease termination difficulties.

Clinical Case: Gary

The following dialogue occurred during one of Gary's last sessions. He was facing an imminent transplant and hoped that the new skills he had learned would give him the needed psychological and emotional strengths required over this next serious course of medical treatment. He had made some important gains over the last few months, and his decision-making skills had improved. Gary now had a stronger sense of confidence and expectation of his own coping ability without the use of alcohol. Additionally, he decreased the frequency with which he negatively interpreted the intentions of others and rarely exhibited angry outbursts. Finally, he had increased the quality of communication with his wife. He now faced a very challenging medical experience. Gary's future goals included plans, when medically stable, to rebuild his marriage with Celia. This session dialogue illustrates an example of the mixed emotions experienced at termination and of the need to apply the problem-solving model toward therapy completion and discharge.

> GARY.   I hope I don't screw up—how many problem-solving failures have you had Doc?
>
> THERAPIST.   Whoa . . . that's a loaded question . . . let's stop and think about what's behind it so that together we can come up with the answer that you are seeking.
>
> GARY.   I just want to know how many failures you've had.
>
> THERAPIST.   Suppose I told you 10 . . . or none . . . or 15 . . . would you have the information that you want right now?
>
> GARY.   No . . . well . . . it's just that I wish we had a little longer to gear up—like it's time for the ball game [the transplant] to begin, and I don't know if I'm in shape yet . . . maybe I'm not done with "spring training."
>
> THERAPIST.   To take your own ball game analogy further, it sounds like you have some concerns that your trainer [the therapist] won't be with you on the field and you want to know how many winners he or she helped prepare for the season. . . . Of course we've talked often about how each person is an individual. Even if I gave you some actual numbers, that would not say too much about how ready *you* are.

GARY.   I'm sorry . . . stupid, huh?

THERAPIST.   You know I'm not going to let you get away with that. During our initial discussions we had, I remember pointing out to you how you had learned to react to fear. Do you remember? Fear led to anger at the other person, which then led to guilt, which then led to putting yourself down—a real spiral of emotions, with very little rational thinking going on to figure out your feelings and begin solving the problem for yourself. We all are more likely to fall back on old habits of emotional reacting and thinking when under stress. The important thing is that we catch ourselves. Because any change is stressful, we can predict that you are under increased stress now—we will be ending working together soon and you will confront the experience of a bone marrow transplant. Quite naturally, you're scared.

GARY.   You got that right!

THERAPIST.   So . . .

GARY.   So . . . STOP and THINK about what's frightening me and do something about it!

THERAPIST.   Sounds good.

GARY.   Well, you said it exactly. I'm getting this transplant and I don't know if I can make it—I mean either actually live through the transplant or make it in terms of my own ways of coping—I just don't know. I wish you could be there with me. I want to know that I'm going to be okay, and I want to know that things are going to be okay with Celia.

THERAPIST.   Knowing that you no longer require meeting with me to know what problem-solving skills to use, what would having me there give you?

GARY.   Someone I could count on to report to about the problems I'm trying to solve—how I'm thinking about them, and to let me know if I'm on the right track. Also, I'm afraid that Celia may not want to work on our relationship if I'm not coming here—I think she needs to know that I am willing to come to a kind of "neutral" place to talk about our problems. We talk better, but we're not there yet . . . you know what I mean?

THERAPIST.   I sure do. I think that you have identified this problem quite clearly. You're feeling apprehensive about facing the transplant and know that you should put your problem-solving skills to work with this issue. Because you're not quite sure if you can successfully cope with all the large and small problems associated with the transplant, you wish that you could be more confident about your new skills and have some way of maximizing your chances for success. However, using problem-solving principles, we can see that having me available at the hospital throughout this experience is only one solution. Can you think of others?

GARY. Yeah . . . probably.

Clinical Commentary

Gary eventually developed the following list of strategies to help keep up with his problem-solving efforts through his transplant experience.

- Teach a friend problem-solving principles and ask for his reaction concerning Gary's management of problems during the transplant.
- Bring problem-solving homework sheets and notebook to the hospital so that he could comprehensively address each skill area when addressing a very difficult problem.
- Teach problem-solving principles to Celia and ask Celia to serve as a problem-solving coach.
- Keep working notes regarding problem-solving efforts and review them as if he were correcting someone else's homework concerning problem description, brainstorming, and selection of alternatives
- Gradually end treatment with successively longer time periods between sessions.
- End treatment soon, but schedule a follow-up session to report on progress after the transplant.
- End problem-solving treatment, but contact a marriage therapist to continue work on the marriage after the recovery from the transplant.
- Hold imaginary therapy sessions and play the role of the therapist in challenging his own ideas and homework.
- Use a tape recorder to complete problem-solving notes when feeling too sick to write things down.

Gary ultimately selected a combination of these alternatives to help the termination process run more smoothly. These included scheduling one posttransplant follow-up session with the problem-solving therapist, bringing homework sheets to the hospital, and discussing a later referral to a marriage therapist with Celia if their relationship did not improve through their own problem-solving attempts.

Gary's final problem-solving session prior to his transplant was focused on making sure his termination plan was in place. These psychological activities replaced the experience of confusion, sadness, fear of failing, and anger at the therapist's absence that had marked his reactions in the previous sessions.

FOLLOW-UP SESSIONS

Similar to Gary, some patients may require booster or follow-up sessions because of new stressors that occur in their lives or ones that are anticipated to occur in the future. For example, patients who come out of remission, have a recurrence, or have difficulty complying with treatment regimens may briefly return to treatment for additional support or coaching. Others may return with a concrete, specific problem that they have identified but believe is too significant to rely solely on their own problem-solving ability without professional feedback. One example is a 36-year-old woman, Jana, who had unprotected sex with her significant other, which resulted in an unplanned pregnancy. Although there were some identified health risks, she was inclined to carry the pregnancy to term. She went through the problem-solving process with her partner but wanted reassurance and validation regarding the rationality of her thinking. Thus, accompanied by her mate, she returned for a series of three problem-solving sessions..

For the majority of individuals who have shown significant improvements in therapy and who are generally satisfied with their treatment, additional sessions are not usually indicated. However, because of the unpredictable nature of cancer and the disease process, it is advisable to conclude treatment with an agreement that the decision to return to therapy can be readdressed if necessary.

Clinical Case Epilogue: Terry

The last time we focused on Terry was at the end of GOA training. With regard to the DM session, she progressed almost effortlessly. In her position as a real estate agent, she frequently used similar strategies of conducting cost–benefit analyses and selecting optimal combinations of solution options when negotiating property sales, amenities, payment plans, and home improvement options with her customers. Likewise, when implementing solutions for problems at work or for most daily hassles, Terry was generally successful.

As previously noted, however, Terry demonstrated a tendency to avoid dealing with problems in general. Yet, she was able to decrease her avoidant behavior in the earlier sessions of therapy by learning new ways to identify problems as they occurred. However, avoidance sometimes interfered with the timely implementation of solution plans directly related to her body-image concerns or communication with her family. Mostly, Terry attributed her difficulties to her diminished self-esteem and absence of an adequate support system. She continued to battle against the negative problem orientation that she had developed during her failed marriage. Despite the occasionally recurring themes of self-doubt, Terry was motivated to make changes in her life. By the end of her weekly therapy sessions, she was responsible for many positive changes in her thinking and in her lifestyle, including improved relations with her parents.

TERRY'S PROBLEM WITH HER COLLEAGUES

Referring to the problem Terry addressed during the GOA session, she recounted the options she had to choose from to cope with her coworkers' and others' stories about cancer victims. Rather than becoming defensive when others told her how "lucky she was to get through it [her diagnosis and treatment]," Terry decided to accept these words literally. She used positive statements both in self-talk and in response to others. She shared parts of conversations with her therapist describing her positive responses such as "Yes, I am very lucky. I am sorry that your friend–family member had a difficult time, but I am happy to be recovering quite well. I am putting the experience behind me and moving on with my life." She would then politely change the conversation or excuse herself if she was uncomfortable with the company. Furthermore, Terry increased the number of positive activities in which she participated during the course of the week. Overall, her mood began to improve.

In accordance with the SIV training, Terry paid attention to the effects of actions and statements. She recorded her own thoughts and feelings that resulted from these positive changes on the Record of Coping Attempts worksheets. Noting the reaction of others, Terry pleasingly found that coworkers and friends from her book club made more effort to spend time with her and invite her to socialize. They also made less mention of her cancer experience, and she no longer felt "pitied." Terry was optimistic that she would be able to overcome the awkwardness she felt at work, and she had less desire to avoid social activities or other people.

SIX MONTHS LATER

Terry returned to her therapist for a follow-up visit 6 months after she had terminated therapy. Over the last several months, many changes continued to occur. Terry had moved out of her parents' home and into a two-bedroom apartment with a college friend who had moved into town. Regaining her financial, social, and emotional independence from her parents had a tremendously positive impact on Terry. She truly felt "lucky to be alive." At times, she struggled with negative thoughts doubting that these positive changes would last. Naturally, she also revisited feelings of sadness or fears of recurrence on occasion. However, her new roommate was very supportive when Terry was feeling depressed or anxious. She also expanded her social support network by entrusting others to become closer to her. Therefore, when Terry felt down or nervous, these moods usually passed fairly quickly.

In the month prior to this follow-up visit with her therapist, Terry decided to devote a portion of her free time to help others with recent diagnoses of breast cancer. She became a volunteer in her local Reach-to-Recovery program that she had found helpful several months prior. Having made many changes in her life, she decided to help others by sharing her experiences. Terry believed that people needed to see others who have survived and who have managed to put their lives back together.

In talking to her therapist, Terry described her returning problem related to body-image concerns. Terry's feelings of uncertainty regarding her appearance resurfaced as a result of a new relationship. After much research and consideration, Terry decided to have reconstructive surgery 1 month after her weekly therapy ended. She told her therapist how pleased she was with the results. Although the scarring remained a constant reminder, she decided that her experience with cancer had positive effects for her also. She explained that these positive effects were evidenced by her renewed self-esteem and positive outlook on life. Recently, however, Terry had begun dating again and believed that she had met a man with whom she was interested in pursuing a relationship. She encountered new fears about intimacy and acceptance, which stemmed from previously unsuccessful relationships, and about her physical changes. However, Terry now believed that she had the resources to overcome her fears by talking to other survivors, relying on her problem-solving skills, and attempting open communication with her new partner when it seemed appropriate. One year ago, Terry would never have attempted to address such complex problems on her own. At the time of her follow-up visit, however, she considered her therapist to be part of her contingency or backup plan if her initial problem-solving efforts did not result in a desirable outcome.

Summary

Practice, practice, practice were the key words underlying the purpose of these last problem-solving sessions. Practice facilitates competence and generalization across problems and over time with new problems. Problem-solving expertise also serves to prevent certain problems from happening in the future. Returning to the saying we had introduced earlier that underlies our philosophy of training—"Give a person a fish, he eats for a day; teach a person to fish, he eats for a lifetime!"—practice helps to increase the likelihood that the patient can now fish in multiple types of environments and catch multiple types of fish. In addition, these practice sessions help reinforce the problem orientation principle that problems are an inevitable part of life, but by using the problem-solving skills that they learned, individuals will now be better equipped to cope with them; for as the famous poet Emily Dickinson stated, "Low as my problem bending, another problem comes."

Key Training Points

- Review goals of PST
- Ask for examples of how these goals have been met
- Reinforce patient's efforts
- Convey your belief in patient's abilities to cope independently
- Discuss thoughts and feelings about ending treatment
- Have patient establish an overall plan to monitor progress made from treatment or use of problem-solving skills
- Discuss option for return to treatment, if indicated

Group Tips

- When group training comes to a close, patients may be offered the same opportunity to return for a refresher session, either for an individual session or as part of a future group, if appropriate.
- Patients can be encouraged, if appropriate, to maintain contact with certain other members to serve as problem-solving coaches.
- Group members can be asked to provide help to each other if termination difficulties arise.

IV | ADAPTATION OF PROBLEM-SOLVING THERAPY FOR CAREGIVER TRAINING

Problem-Solving Education for Family Caregivers of Cancer Patients

11

Overview

Family members and friends who care for cancer patients at home are becoming increasingly important in the provision of health care. They are responsible for managing care in the home, including monitoring the illness, carrying out prescribed treatments, informing health-care professionals when problems arise, and providing emotional and social support for the patient. With the increase in the number of people living with cancer, more and more family members are having to take on these responsibilities. In addition, as a result of changes in the health-care system represented by shorter hospitalizations and more reliance on outpatient care, tasks, which until recently have only been assigned to trained, supervised health-care personnel, are being shifted to family caregivers.

Unfortunately, family caregivers who are assuming these responsibilities are often uninformed about what they should do, unskilled in carrying out medical duties, and emotionally unprepared as well. As a result, there is significant risk of compromising the quality of patient care and of causing significant caregiver burden and morbidity. Studies of spouses of seriously ill patients have reported eating disorders, sleep disturbances, anxiety, and depression because of the stresses of caregiving (Kristjanson & Ashercroft, 1994; Oberst, Thomas, Gass, & Ward, 1989). If these problems are to be controlled, family caregivers must be taught how to cope with their new responsibilities. We suggest that our problem-solving model offers an ideal approach to help caregivers deal with such responsibilities, as well as how to access and use relevant expert information about the cancer and associated difficulties. In this final chapter, we describe the adaption of the problem-solving principles in developing a model for caregivers of cancer patients. This protocol teaches them how to be more effective caregivers, as well as serving as a means to minimize the burden and distress often associated with caregiving responsibilities.

A Problem-Solving Model of Caregiver Training

Family caregivers need to know *what* to do, *when* to do it, and at a level appropriate for their backgrounds, they need to understand *why* they should do it. The information should be understandable by individuals without training in biology, psychology, and medicine. Furthermore, information should be organized in terms of problems, such that it can efficiently be accessed for solving caregiving difficulties. Most patient education materials are not organized in terms of problems. Rather, they typically involve loosely organized discussions of medical procedures and symptoms. What is needed is information structured around the steps that can be taken to solve specific problems.

Our work in developing educational materials to support problem-solving activities among caregivers of cancer patients indicates that the following types of information are needed to solve caregiving problems while working cooperatively with health-care professionals (Houts, Nezu, Nezu, & Bucher, 1996):

1. An understanding of the problem at a level appropriate for caregivers' backgrounds and training (i.e., what is the problem, who is most likely to have it, when they have it, what kinds of things can be done to help, and what are realistic goals when dealing with the problem);
2. Knowing when to get professional help (e.g., when to call immediately, when to call during office hours, what information to have when the caregiver calls, and what to say);
3. Knowing what family caregivers can do to help (i.e., to deal with, as well as prevent, problems);
4. Possible obstacles (i.e., misinformation or obstacles that can interfere with carrying out the plan and how to deal with them); and

5. How to carry out and adjust the plan (e.g., how to check on whether the caregiver is making progress, how fast to expect change, and what to do if it the plan is not working).

Often medical interventions appear to have little or no effect in the short run, but they do have long-term benefits. Therefore, the information given to family caregivers should also include explanations of the kinds of events that indicate progress and in what time periods change may be expected.

We have found that when such problem-solving information is organized in manual form, it can facilitate communication between medical staff and family caregivers and can help professionals monitor the care given at home. When both staff and family caregivers have copies of the manuals, they can easily communicate what is being done and identify the areas in which problems are occurring. The manuals can also give family caregivers and patients a sense of control over their problems, allowing them to develop plans in advance, before problems occur or become severe.

TRAINING PATIENTS AND FAMILY CAREGIVERS IN EFFECTIVE PROBLEM-SOLVING STRATEGIES

Information, however, is not enough. Family caregivers need to learn to use information in the context of an orderly problem-solving approach to caregiving. This is what health-care professionals learn, and because the responsibilities given to patients and caregivers for managing care at home are in many cases equivalent, they need to learn these same problem-solving skills for their caregiving. Such training can increase self-confidence, as family caregivers are often intimidated by health-care professionals and need reassurance that their problem-solving activities are sanctioned.

Fortunately, there is evidence that nonprofessionals can learn problem-solving skills and that they can derive benefits from such training (see chapter 2). The conceptual model for problem-solving education, which we have recently developed (Houts et al., 1996), adapts the concepts used in PST (i.e., problem orientation, problem definition and formulation, generation of alternatives, decision making, and solution implementation and verification) to the special needs of family caregivers coping with serious illness, such as cancer. It has four major components, as summarized by the acronym *COPE* (i.e., *C*reativity, *O*ptimism, *P*lanning, and *E*xpert Information). Listed in the following paragraphs are the definitions of these components and their relationship to the other components in PST.

The *Creativity* component of the problem-solving education model adapts the generation-of-alternatives process in the PST model to the special needs of coping with physical illness. It is important, especially when the patient's health can be affected, to follow directions from health-care professionals to solve problems (e.g., high fever or suicide). However, overcoming obstacles in carrying out medical management (e.g., lack of cooperation from other family members) provides many opportunities and challenges for which creativity is essential. To implement the creativity component, the problem solver steps back from the situation and views it from a new perspective to develop creative solutions. This not only increases the likelihood of successfully overcoming obstacles, but it also has important psychological consequences as well. Viewing the problem from new perspectives helps to break negative thought patterns and supports expectations that the problem is solvable.

The *Optimism* component of this model addresses the cognitive and emotional aspects of problem solving and includes the orientation component of the PST model that refers to the attitudes and expectations that a person has regarding problems in living and the motivation to carry out the problem-solving steps. In coping with a serious illness, optimism should be tempered with realism, as it is in the PST model. People with serious illnesses and their families need realistic optimism, which recognizes the seriousness of the problem and, at the same time, includes the expectation that something can be done to deal with the problem. Setting realistic goals is a key part of optimism because this focuses attention on goals that are achievable with reasonable effort and, therefore, justifies positive expectations. Optimism, in this model, also includes interpersonal skills that enable patients and caregivers to communicate positively and to cooperate in the planning.

Planning is the central component of problem solving. Although planning medical treatments is done largely by health-care professionals in consultation with the patient, families and patients must develop plans for carrying out medical instructions and for dealing with most psychosocial problems related to the illness. These plans include the following rational problem-solving skills: obtaining complete information, separating facts from conjecture, specifying who will do what and when, and carrying out and monitoring the plan. Developing a plan reduces uncertainty by specifying what will be done under what circumstances. Planning can also lead to better problem resolution, which ultimately leads to less distress and better overall coping.

The *Expert Information* component is an addition to the PST model discussed throughout this text and includes obtaining guidance from health-care professionals for dealing with physical and psychosocial problems that are due to cancer and its treatment. Expert information empowers patients and family caregivers by enabling them to develop effective plans for solving problems related to the illness. It has important psychological consequences as well. This information provides patients and caregivers with a sense of control by clearly explaining what they can do. It also defines the limits of what they need to do, which is helpful when dealing with problems for the first time. Uncertainty about "Have I done everything I can?" may result in patients and family caregivers pushing themselves beyond reasonable limits. Properly organized expert information can give people an understanding of the limits of what is expected of them.

TEACHING PROBLEM SOLVING TO FAMILY CAREGIVERS THROUGH CASE EXAMPLES

We have found case studies to be an excellent way to teach caregivers how to use the COPE problem-solving techniques. Training through cases is widely used in training health-care professionals to solve problems—we have found that they are effective in training family caregivers as well. Family caregivers are very interested in how other caregivers solved their problems and, therefore, respond positively to learning through this approach. Once caregivers have developed plans for other people's problems, they can adapt those plans to their own situations.

An important advantage of teaching through case examples is that the stories engage the interest of caregivers and demonstrate the relevance of what is being taught. This is especially important in teaching adults who have many competing demands for their time and energy. Another advantage of case teaching is that caregivers can see how the different problem-solving elements interact and support one another. They also provide an opportunity to demonstrate or model how patients and caregivers should approach their problem solving, including how to work cooperatively with health-care professionals.

THE PREPARED FAMILY CAREGIVER COURSE

The following is an example of how problem-solving training can be accomplished by utilizing case examples. This program, entitled the *Prepared Family Caregiver Course*, has recently been implemented and field tested in central Pennsylvania. The course materials consist of an instructor's manual, a videotape, and, for each participant, a copy of the *Home Care Guide for Cancer* (Houts et al., 1994). This guide serves as a problem-solving manual and includes the expert information needed to solve 21 common problems related to caring for a cancer patient (e.g., fever, fatigue, bleeding, communication, and depression). The course is designed to be led by a team consisting of a health professional (usually a nurse) and a human service professional, such as a psychologist, social worker, counselor, or clergy person. Because the didactic material is on videotape, the group can be led by professionals who are not necessarily experienced teachers or specialists in cancer care. The interactions among participants are the core of the program and the context within which the important learning takes place. The videotapes are used to present standardized information that the group uses in its interactions. Each session of the course is divided into three segments, as described next.

Introduction and Explanation of the COPE Problem-Solving Techniques

The COPE techniques are explained on the videotape by telling a story of how a family caregiver solved a difficult caregiving problem. The story is told as a "play," with the principal characters speaking their parts. After the story is told, the COPE concepts are introduced to explain what has occurred. This segment ends with participants discussing how they have solved caregiving problems and have used the COPE techniques in their lives.

Practice Using the COPE Techniques to Develop a Plan for Solving a Caregiving Problem Presented as a Case

The second segment consists of a story that is organized to allow participants to practice each of the COPE techniques. The story is told on video, with pauses for participants to find expert information, think up creative ideas, develop an orderly plan, and discuss how the plan should be presented to the cancer patient in a way that shows understanding, as well as hope and optimism.

Develop a Plan for Solving Participants' Caregiving Problems

Having completed a plan for a caregiving problem, participants then use what they have learned and develop a similar plan for themselves. They do this in pairs to ensure that each participant has an opportunity to explain and receive feedback from another person regarding his or her plan, thereby avoiding the danger of having this important part of the course dominated by a few "talkative" persons. The segment ends with participants sharing plans with the group as a whole and seeing a video segment that summarizes what has been learned in a given session.

Evaluation Data From the Prepared Family Caregiver Course

Although it was designed primarily for family caregivers, the prepared family caregiver course has attracted a much broader audience. Family caregivers, hospice volunteers, home health aides and nurses, and individuals with cancer have completed the course. Written evaluations indicate a high level of satisfaction and interest in using the information and problem-solving skills that were taught.

To assess the impact of the course with specific regard to caregivers of cancer patients, we recently conducted a small pilot evaluation. Specifically, in follow-up interviews with 36 participants, who were caring for someone with cancer at the time of the course, these participants were asked how they had used the course information and materials in their caregiving. Two sets of questions were of particular interest: (a) how many caregivers used the plans developed during the course and (b) how many used the *Home Care Guide for Cancer* in dealing with subsequent caregiving problems. Forty-nine percent reported using the plans that they had developed during the course in their caregiving, and 67% said they had used the *Guide* to manage specific caregiving problems after the course. Many who had not used the book or the plans said that it was because the person with cancer either died or went into remission shortly after attending the course.

After the course, more than half of these cancer patient caregivers reported that they had at least skimmed all 23 chapters in the *Guide* whether or not the person with cancer had experienced the specific problem addressed by a given chapter. The entire sample reported reading an average of 16.5 total chapters. Data further indicated that topics related to physical problems were read as frequently as those concerning social or emotional problems.

Because the course emphasizes the value of proactive problem solving, we were also interested in whether course participants had developed plans before the problem became a crisis. We found that 19 of the 22 people who had read the *Home Care Guide* did so prior to their problems becoming crises, whereas 14 said that they had developed conscious plans for how they would go about dealing with problems. These results indicate that many of the attendees used the problem-solving information and strategies proactively as taught in the prepared family caregiver course. Rigorous experimental–control group comparisons are planned in the near future to determine the extent to which the course and follow-up support for problem solving actually change behaviors and feelings of competence in carrying out the role of family caregiver for this population.

Need for Continuing Support for Problem-Solving Activities

Although the evaluation results are encouraging, they deal only with the immediate effects of the course. It has become clear in implementing this program that ongoing support for problem solving is important if family caregivers are to continue using problem-solving principles over time. Support can come from several sources, including health-care professionals, family caregiver support groups, and newly available technology in the form of electronic bulletin board systems.

SUPPORT FROM HEALTH-CARE PROFESSIONALS

If patients and families are to invest time and effort in developing and carrying out orderly plans, health-care professionals involved in the patients' care must give continuing support for their problem-solving efforts. Fortunately, a model exists for how this can be done. Bone marrow transplant programs routinely teach caregiving skills to patients and families, which they use outside of the hospital. Health-care professionals have found that patients and families take these responsibilities seriously when (a) they are told at the outset that this is an expected and required part of the program; (b) staff emphasizes the importance of the responsibilities for the patients' health; (c) all members of the health team support the need for the patients' and families' participation; and (d) performance is assessed continuously.

These same strategies can be used in programs to teach and support problem-solving efforts to patients and their family caregivers. The problem-solving course can be presented as an essential part of the treatment program and can be scheduled along with tests and medical procedures. After completion of the three training sessions, treatment staff can encourage and provide support to patients and the family caregivers by using the COPE problem-solving strategies and the *Home Care Guide*. This support can be integrated into the staff's routine interactions with patients, and, thus, the patients' require little additional staff time.

PROBLEM-SOLVING SUPPORT GROUPS

Support and encouragement from other family caregivers can also play an important role in supporting problem-solving activities. We have observed that family caregivers are very interested in how other caregivers have dealt with problems that they are experiencing, and they are often reassured and comforted by talking with other family caregivers. A problem-solving support group allows caregivers to give and receive emotional support, to share problem-solving techniques, and to help one another develop problem-solving plans for difficult problems.

Support groups are usually organized as face-to-face meetings. For those who attend, such meetings are supportive and helpful. Unfortunately, attendance is often small. This is because of competing demands of caregiving, difficulty in arranging transportation, and reluctance to exposing oneself to strangers. Fortunately, some recent technological innovations can help in overcoming these barriers. Internet-type bulletin boards allow people with computers to communicate without the problems of leaving home and of exposing one's identity to others. CHESS (Comprehensive Health Enhancement Support System) is an example of such a program designed to allow communication among people dealing with breast cancer and other illnesses (Gustafson et al., 1993). The CHESS program also contains information about different aspects of breast cancer, as well as a decision-making module that guides women in making decisions about their treatment.

The Telepractice program is similar to the CHESS program, but it uses a touch-tone phone instead of a personal computer (Alemi et al., 1996). Participants in the Telepractice system use the touch-tone phones to navigate the bulletin board system and leave voice messages, rather than messages typed from a computer keyboard. The program is managed by a computer that stores and plays messages as directed by signals from the users' phones. The Telepractice system can be used by anyone capable of using a touch-tone telephone and has the advantage of allowing participants to communicate by voice, which is more personal, showing emotion more clearly than typed messages. As with other bulletin-board programs, messages are posted under topics, and listeners can browse the list and choose to make contributions at their discretion. Participants can also ask questions and receive answers from experts, as well as share information and support one another. The limitations of the Telepractice system, in comparison to computer-based programs such as CHESS, are that it is less feasible to provide access to books or other lengthy sources of information and it is not possible to show pictures or graphics.

Both the telephone and computer-based bulletin boards have the potential for supporting family caregiver problem-solving efforts. These boards can provide expert information that caregivers need, and, as in the CHESS program, they can include programs that guide the user in developing plans. Also, the question-and-answer format and the discussion group format provide opportunities for professionals to encourage and support the use of an orderly problem-solving approach to caregiving problems. Telephone and computer-based bulletin boards are also efficient uses of professional time because professionals can listen to and respond to questions or discussion at their convenience and because receiving and sending messages are managed automatically by computer programs. We are currently in the process of developing and evaluating both types of problem-solving programs for caregivers of cancer patients.

Conclusion

The shift of health care from the hospital to the home has markedly increased duties and responsibilities that family caregivers must assume and has made them members of the health-care team. These family members must solve a wide range of caregiving problems while working cooperatively with health-care professionals. To accomplish this, family caregivers need information organized to support problem-solving efforts and they need training in how to apply an orderly problem-solving process to caregiving problems—the same as health-care professionals do.

To meet this psychosocial need, we have developed the *Home Care Guide for Cancer*, a manual-based training protocol specific to cancer caregivers. The problem-solving model previously delineated in this book has been adapted into the COPE format. Using this approach, we further developed the prepared family caregiver course, which utilizes this guidebook, in addition to a series of videotapes that train cancer caregivers in the problem-solving model in which case examples are used. Preliminary evaluation of this approach underscores its potential effectiveness.

For problem-solving education to affect caregiving behavior in the home, there must be ongoing support from health-care professionals and from other family caregivers. Additional support can come from the creative use of technology, as in computer or voice bulletin boards, in which answers to patients' and families' questions are treated as opportunities to teach and support problem-solving activities.

References

Alemi F., Stephens, R. C., Mosavel, M., Ghadiri, A., Krishnaswany, J., & Thakkar, H. (1996). Electronic self help and support groups: A voice bulletin board. *Medical Care Supplement: Computer Services to Patients' Homes Through Their Telephones, 34,* 10532–10544.

American Cancer Society. (1997). *Cancer facts and figures—1997.* Atlanta, GA: Author.

American Psychiatric Association. (1994). *Diagnostic and statistical manual of mental disorders* (4th ed.). Washington, DC: Author.

Arean, P. A., Perri, M. G., Nezu, A. M., Schein, R. L., Christopher, F., & Joseph, T. X. (1993). Comparative effectiveness of social problem-solving therapy and reminiscence therapy as treatments for depression in older adults. *Journal of Consulting and Clinical Psychology, 61,* 1003–1010.

Arnkoff, D. B. (1983). Common and specific factors in cognitive therapy. In M. J. Lambert (Ed.), *Psychotherapy and patient relationships* (pp. 85–125). Homewood, IL: Dorsey Press.

Bandura, A. (1977). Self-efficacy: Toward a unifying theory of behavior change. *Psychological Review, 84,* 191–215.

Baron, R. M., & Kenny, D. A. (1986). The moderator–mediator variable distinction in social psychological research: Conceptual, strategic, and statistical considerations. *Journal of Personality and Social Psychology, 51,* 1173–1182.

Baumgardner, A. H., Heppner, P. P., & Arkin, R. M. (1986). The role of causal attribution in personal problem solving. *Journal of Personality and Social Psychology, 50,* 636–643.

Beck, A. T., Kovacs, M., & Weissman, A. (1975). Hopelessness and suicidal behavior: An overview. *Journal of the American Medical Association, 234,* 1146–1149.

Beck, A. T., Rush, A. J., Shaw, B. F., & Emery, G. (1979). *Cognitive therapy of depression: A treatment manual.* New York: Guilford Press.

Beck, A. T., Ward, C. H., Mendelson, M., Mock, J., & Erbaugh, J. (1961). An inventory for measuring depression. *Archives of General Psychiatry, 5,* 462–467.

Bloom, B. S., & Broder, L. J. (1950). *Problem-solving processes of college students.* Chicago: University of Chicago Press.

Bolund, C. (1985). Suicide and cancer: I. Demographic and social characteristics of cancer patients in Sweden, 1973–1976. *Journal of Psychosocial Oncology, 3,* 31–52.

Bradshaw, W. H. (1993). Coping-skills training versus a problem-solving approach with schizophrenic patients. *Hospital and Community Psychiatry, 44,* 1102–1104.

Breitbart, W. (1990). Suicide. In J. C. Holland & J. H. Rowland (Eds.), *Handbook of psychooncology* (pp. 291–299). New York: Oxford University Press.

Byrd, B. L. (1983). Late effects of treatment of cancer in children. *Pediatric Annals, 12,* 450–460.

Cassileth, B. R., Walsh, W. P., & Lusk, E. J. (1988). Psychosocial correlates of cancer survival: A subsequent report 3 to 8 years after cancer diagnosis. *Journal of Clinical Oncology, 6,* 1753–1759.

Cella, D. F., Tulsky, D. S., Gray, G., Sarafran, B., Linn, E., Bonomi, A., Silberman, M., Yellen, S. B., Winicour, P., & Brannon, J. (1993). The Functional Assessment of Cancer Therapy Scale: Development and validation of the general measure. *Journal of Clinical Oncology, 11,* 570–579.

Chang, E. C., & D'Zurilla, T. J. (1996). Relations between problem orientation and optimism, pessimism, and trait affectivity: A construct validation study. *Behaviour Therapy and Research, 34,* 185–194.

Cormier, W. H., Otani, A., & Cormier, S. (1986). The effects of problem-solving training on two problem-solving tasks. *Cognitive Therapy and Research, 10,* 95–108.

Dahlstrom, W. G., & Welsh, G. S. (1960). *An MMPI handbook.* Minneapolis: University of Minnesota Press.

Deaner, S. L., Nezu, A. M., & Nezu, C. M. (1997, August). *Problem-solving ability, optimism, and distress.* Paper presented at the 105th Annual Convention of the American Psychological Association, Chicago.

Derogatis, L. R. (1986). *Derogatis Interview of Sexual Function—Self-report.* Baltimore, MD: Clinical Psychometric Research.

Derogatis, L. R., & Spencer, P. M. (1982). *The Brief Symptom Inventory: Administration, scoring and procedures manual.* Baltimore, MD: Clinical Psychometric Research.

Dewey, J. (1910). *How we think.* Princeton, NJ: Princeton University Press.

DiGiuseppe, R., Simon, K. S., McGowan, L., & Gardner, F. (1990). A comparative outcome study of four cognitive therapies in the treatment of social anxiety. *Journal of Rational–Emotive and Cognitive–Behavior Therapy, 8,* 129–146.

Dreher, H. (1997). The scientific and moral imperative for broad-based psychosocial interventions for cancer. *Advances: The Journal of Mind–Body Health, 13,* 38–49.

Dugas, M. J., Letarte, H., Rheaume, J., Freeston, M. H., & Ladoucer, R. (1995). Worry and problem solving: Evidence of a specific relationship. *Cognitive Therapy and Research, 19,* 109–120.

Dunkel-Schetter, C., Feinstein, L. G., Taylor, S. E., & Falke, R. L. (1992).

Patterns of coping with cancer. *Health Psychology, 11*, 79–87.

D'Zurilla, T. J., & Goldfried, M. R. (1971). Problem-solving and behavior modification. *Journal of Abnormal Psychology, 78*, 107–126.

D'Zurilla, T. J., & Nezu, A. (1980). A study of the generation-of-alternatives process in social problem solving. *Cognitive Therapy and Research, 4*, 67–76.

D'Zurilla, T. J., & Nezu, A. (1982). Social problem solving in adults. In P. C. Kendall (Ed.), *Advances in cognitive–behavioral research and therapy* (Vol. 1, pp. 202–274). New York: Academic Press.

D'Zurilla, T. J., & Nezu, A. M. (1990). Development and preliminary evaluation of the Social Problem-Solving Inventory (SPSI). *Psychological Assessment: A Journal of Consulting and Clinical Psychology, 2*, 156–163.

D'Zurilla, T. J., & Nezu, A. M. (in press). *Problem-solving therapy* (2nd ed.). New York: Springer.

D'Zurilla, T. J., Nezu, A. M., & Maydeu-Olivares, A. (in press). *Manual for the Social Problem-Solving Inventory—Revised (SPSI–R)*. North Tonawanda, NY: Multi-Health Systems.

Edgar, L., Rosberger, Z., & Nowlis, D. (1992). Coping with cancer during the first year after diagnosis: Assessment and intervention. *Cancer, 69*, 817–828.

Edwards, W., Lindman, H., & Phillips, L. D. (1965). Emerging technologies for making decisions. In T. M. Newcomb (Ed.), *New directions in psychology* (pp. 291–324). New York: Holt, Rinehart & Winston.

Elliott, T. R., & Johnson, M. O. (1995, August). *Social problem solving and acceptance of disability*. Paper presented at the 103rd Annual Convention of the American Psychological Association, New York.

Elliott, T. R., Sherwin, E., Harkins, S., & Marmarosh, C. (1995). Self-appraised problem-solving ability, affective states, and psychological distress. *Journal of Counseling Psychology, 42*, 105–115.

Elliott, T. R., & Shewchuk, R. (in press). Problem-solving therapy for family caregivers of persons with severe physical disabilities. In C. Radnitz (Ed.), *Cognitive–behavioral interventions for persons with disabilities*. New York: Jason Aronson.

Elliott, T. R., Shewchuk, R. M., Richards, J. S., Palmatier, A. D., & Margolis, K. (1997, April). *Social problem solving and adjustment of caregivers of persons with recent onset spinal cord injury*. Paper presented at annual meeting of the Society of Behavioral Medicine, San Francisco.

Ellis, A. (1985). *Overcoming resistance: Rationale–emotive therapy with difficult clients*. New York: Springer.

Ewart, C. K. (1990). A social problem-solving approach to behavior change in coronary heart disease. In S. A. Schumaker, E. B. Schron, J. K. Ockene, C. T. Parker, J. L. Probstfield, & J. M. Wolle (Eds.), *The handbook of health behavior change* (pp. 153–190). New York: Springer.

Fawzy, F. I., Cousins, N., Fawzy, N., Kemeny, M., Elashoff, R., & Morton, D. (1990). A structured psychiatric intervention for cancer patients: Changes over time in methods of coping and affective disturbance. *Archives of General Psychiatry, 47*, 720–725.

Foley, K. M., & Sundaresen, N. (1985). The management of cancer pain.

In V. T. DeVita, S. Hellman, & S. A. Rosenberg (Eds.), *Cancer: Principles and practices of oncology* (2nd ed., pp. 1940–1961). Philadelphia: Lippincott.

Fox, B. (1983). Current theory of psychogenic effects on cancer incidence and prognosis. *Journal of Psychosocial Oncology, 1,* 17–31.

Fox, B. H., Stanek, S. C., Boyd, S. C., & Flannery, J. T. (1982). Suicide rates among cancer patients in Connecticut. *Journal of Chronic Diseases, 35,* 85–100.

Garcia, H. B., & Lee, P. C. Y. (1989). Knowledge about cancer and use of health care services among Hispanic and Asian–American older adults. *Journal of Psychosocial Oncology, 6,* 157–177.

Godshall, F., & Elliott, T. R. (in press). Behavioral correlates of self-appraised problem-solving ability: Problem-solving skills and health compromising behaviors. *Journal of Applied Social Psychology.*

Goldfried, M. R., & D'Zurilla, T. J. (1969). A behavior-analytic model for assessing competence. In C. D. Spielberger (Ed.), *Current topics in clinical and community psychology* (Vol. 1, pp. 151–196). New York: Academic Press.

Gotlib, I. H., & Asarnow, R. F. (1979). Interpersonal and impersonal problem-solving skills in mildly and moderately depressed university students. *Journal of Consulting and Clinical Psychology, 47,* 86–95.

Greenwald, H. (1975). Humor in psychotherapy. *Journal of Contemporary Psychotherapy, 7,* 113–116.

Gustafson, D., Wise, M., McTavish, F., Taylor, J., Wolberg, W., Stewart, J., Smalley, R. V., & Bosworth, K. (1993). Development and pilot evaluation of a computer-based support system for women with breast cancer. *Journal of Psychosocial Oncology, 11,* 69–93.

Hamilton, M. (1960). A rating scale for depression. *Journal of Neurology, Neurosurgery, and Psychiatry, 23,* 56–62.

Hamilton, M. (1967). Development of a rating scale for primary depressive illness. *British Journal of Social and Clinical Psychology, 6,* 278–296.

Hansen, D. J., St. Lawrence, J. S., & Christoff, K. A. (1985). Effects of interpersonal problem-solving training with chronic aftercare patients on problem-solving component skills and effectiveness of solutions. *Journal of Consulting and Clinical Psychology, 53,* 167–174.

Heppner, P. P., & Anderson, W. P. (1985). The relationship between problem-solving self-appraisal and psychological adjustment. *Cognitive Therapy and Research, 9,* 415–427.

Heppner, P. P., Baumgardner, A. H., & Jackson, J. (1985). The relationship between problem-solving self-appraisal, depression, and attributional style: Are they related? *Cognitive Therapy and Research, 9,* 105–113.

Heppner, P. P., Hibel, J. H., Neal, G. W., Weinstein, C. L., & Rabinowitz, F. E. (1982). Personal problem solving: A descriptive study of individual differences. *Journal of Counseling Psychology, 29,* 580–590.

Heppner, P. P., Kampa, M., & Brunning, L. (1987). The relationship between problem-solving self-appraisal and indices of physical and psychological health. *Cognitive Therapy and Research, 11,* 155–168.

Heppner, P. P., Reeder, B. L., & Larson, L. M. (1983). Cognitive variables associated with personal problem-solving appraisal: Implications for counseling. *Journal of Counseling Psychology, 30,* 537–545.

Hinton, J. (1972). Psychiatric consultation in fatal illness. *Proceedings of the Royal Society of Medicine, 65,* 29–32.

Holland, J. C. (1982). Psychological aspects of cancer. In J. F. Holland & E. Frei, III (Eds.), *Cancer medicine* (2nd ed., pp. 1175–1203). Philadelphia: Lea & Febiger.

Holland, J. C. (1990). Historical overview. In J. C. Holland & J. H. Rowland (Eds.), *Handbook of psychooncology* (pp. 3–12). New York: Oxford University Press.

Holland, J. C., & Rowland, J. H. (Eds.). (1990). *Handbook of psychooncology.* New York: Oxford University Press.

Houts, P. S., Nezu, A. M., Nezu, C. M., & Bucher, J. A. (1996). A problem-solving model of family caregiving for cancer patients. *Patient Education and Counseling, 27,* 63–73.

Houts, P. S., Nezu, A. M., Nezu, C. M., Bucher, J. A., & Lipton, A. (Eds.). (1994). *Home care guide for cancer.* Philadelphia: American College of Physicians.

Houts, P. S., Yasko, J., Kahn, S. B., Schelzel, G., & Marconi, K. (1986). Unmet psychological, social and economic needs of persons with cancer in Pennsylvania. *Cancer, 58,* 2355–2361.

Hussian, R. A., & Lawrence, P. S. (1981). Social reinforcement of activity and problem-solving training in the treatment of institutional-ized elderly patients. *Cognitive Therapy and Research, 5,* 57–69.

Jacobsen, P. B., & Holland, J. C. (1991). The stress of cancer: Psychological responses to diagnosis and treatment. In C. L. Cooper & M. Watson (Eds.), *Cancer and stress: Psychological, biological and coping studies* (pp. 147–169). Chichester, England: Wiley.

Jahoda, M. (1953). The meaning of psychological health. *Social Casework, 34,* 349–354.

Jamison, R. N., Burish, T. G., & Wallston, K. A. (1987). Psychogenic factors in predicting survival of breast cancer patients. *Journal of Clinical Oncology, 5,* 768–772.

Jannoun, L., Munby, M., Catalan, J., & Gelder, M. (1980). A home-based treatment program for agoraphobia: Replication and controlled evaluation. *Behavior Therapy, 11,* 294–305.

Kanfer, F. H. (1970). Self-regulation: Research, issues, and speculations. In C. Neuringer & J. L. Michael (Eds.), *Behavior modification in clinical psychology* (pp. 351–389). New York: Appleton-Century-Crofts.

Kant, G. L., D'Zurilla, T. J., & Maydeu-Olivares, A. (1997). Social problem solving as a mediator of stress-related depression and anxiety in middle-aged and elderly community residents. *Cognitive Therapy and Research, 21,* 73–96.

Kendall, P. C., & Braswell, L. (1985). *Cognitive–behavioral therapy for impulsive children.* New York: Guilford Press.

Kristjanson, L. J., & Ashercroft, T. (1994). The family's cancer journey: A literature review. *Cancer Nursing, 17,* 1–17.

Kuhlman, T. L. (1984). *Humor and psychotherapy*. Homewood, IL: Dow Jones-Irwin.

Kunkel, E. J. S., Woods, C. M., Rodgers, C., & Myers, R. E. (1997). Consultations for "maladaptive denial of illness" in patients with cancer: Psychiatric disorders that result in noncompliance. *Psychooncology, 6*, 139–149.

Lazarus, R. S., & Folkman, S. (1984). *Stress, appraisal, and coping*. New York: Springer.

Lerner, M. S., & Clum, G. A. (1990). Treatment of suicide ideators: A problem-solving approach. *Behavior Therapy, 21*, 403–411.

Levine, P., Silberfarb, P. M., & Lipowski, Z. J. (1978). Mental disorders in cancer patients. *Cancer, 42*, 1385–1391.

Locke, B. Z., & Regier, D. A. (1985). Prevalence of selected mental disorders. In C. A. Taube & S. A. Barrett (Eds.), *Mental health United States 1985* (pp. 1–6). Rockville, MD: National Institute of Mental Health.

Magura, S., Kang, S. Y., & Shapiro, J. L. (1994). Outcomes of intensive AIDS education for male adolescent drug users in jail. *Journal of Adolescent Health, 15*, 457–463.

Mahoney, M. J., & Thoresen, C. E. (1974). *Self-control: Power to the person*. Monterey, CA: Brooks/Cole.

Maier, N. R. F., & Hoffman, L. R. (1964). Financial incentives and group decisions in motivating change. *Journal of Social Psychology, 64*, 369–378.

Marks, D. I., Crilley, P., Nezu, C. M., & Nezu, A. M. (1996). Sexual dysfunction prior to high dose chemother-apy and bone marrow transplantation. *Bone Marrow Transplantation, 17*, 595–599.

Massie, M. J. (1990). Anxiety, panic, and phobias. In J. C. Holland & J. H. Rowland (Eds.), *Handbook of psychooncology* (pp. 300–309). New York: Oxford University Press.

Massie, M. J., & Holland, J. C. (1988). Consultation and liaison issues in cancer care. *Psychiatric Medicine, 5*, 343–359.

Maydeu-Olivares, A., & D'Zurilla, T. J. (1996). A factor-analytic study of the Social Problem Solving Inventory: An integration of theory and data. *Cognitive Therapy and Research, 20*, 115–133.

McDowell, I., & Newell, C. (1996). *Measuring health: A guide to rating scales and questionnaires* (2nd ed.). Oxford, England: Oxford University Press.

McNair, D. M., Lorr, M., & Droppleman, L. F. (1992). *Manual for the Profile of Mood States*. San Diego, CA: EDITS.

Meyerowitz, B. E. (1983). Postmastectomy coping strategies and quality of life. *Health Psychology, 2*, 117–132.

Monroe, S. M. (1983). Major and minor life events as predictors of psychological distress: Further issues and findings. *Journal of Behavioral Medicine, 6*, 189–205.

Mooney, R. L., & Gordon, L. V. (1950). *Manual: The Mooney Problem Checklist*. New York: Psychological Corporation.

Murphy, G. P., Morris, L. B., & Lange, D. (1997). *Informed decisions: The complete book of cancer diagnosis, treatment, and recovery*. New York: Viking.

Mynors-Wallis, L. M., Gath, D. H., Lloyd-Thomas, A. R., & Tomlinson,

D. (1995). Randomised controlled trial comparing problem solving treatment with amitryptyline and placebo for major depression in primary care. *British Medical Journal, 310*, 441–445.

Neal, G. W., & Heppner, P. P. (1982, March). *Personality correlates of effective problem solving*. Paper presented at the annual meeting of the American Personnel and Guidance Association, Detroit, MI.

Nezu, A. M. (1985). Differences in psychological distress between effective and ineffective problem solvers. *Journal of Counseling Psychology, 32*, 135–138.

Nezu, A. M. (1986a). Cognitive appraisal of problem-solving effectiveness: Relation to depression and depressive symptoms. *Journal of Clinical Psychology, 42*, 42–48.

Nezu, A. M. (1986b). The effects of stress from current problems: Comparison to major life events. *Journal of Clinical Psychology, 42*, 847–852.

Nezu, A. M. (1986c). Efficacy of a social problem-solving therapy approach for unipolar depression. *Journal of Consulting and Clinical Psychology, 54*, 196–202.

Nezu, A. M. (1986d). Negative life stress and anxiety: Problem solving as a moderator variable. *Psychological Reports, 58*, 279–283.

Nezu, A. M. (1987). A problem-solving formulation of depression: A literature review and proposal of a pluralistic model. *Clinical Psychology Review, 7*, 122–144.

Nezu, A. M., & Carnevale, G. J. (1987). Interpersonal problem solving and coping reactions of Vietnam veterans with posttraumatic stress disorder. *Journal of Abnormal Psychology, 96*, 155–157.

Nezu, A., & D'Zurilla, T. J. (1979). An experimental evaluation of the decision making process in social problem solving. *Cognitive Therapy and Research, 3*, 269–277.

Nezu, A., & D'Zurilla, T. J. (1981a). Effects of problem definition and formulation on decision making in the social problem-solving process. *Behavior Therapy, 12*, 100–106.

Nezu, A., & D'Zurilla, T. J. (1981b). Effects of problem definition and formulation on the generation-of-alternatives process in social problem solving. *Cognitive Therapy and Research, 5*, 265–271.

Nezu, A. M., & D'Zurilla, T. J. (1989). Social problem solving and negative affective states. In P. C. Kendall & D. Watson (Eds.), *Anxiety and depression: Distinctive and overlapping features* (pp. 285–315). New York: Academic Press.

Nezu, A. M., Kalmar, K., Ronan, G. F., & Clavijo, A. (1986). Attributional correlates of depression: An interactional model including problem solving. *Behavior Therapy, 17*, 50–56.

Nezu, A. M., & Nezu, C. M. (Eds.). (1989). *Clinical decision making in behavior therapy: A problem-solving perspective*. Champaign, IL: Research Press.

Nezu, A. M., & Nezu, C. M. (1998, February). *Problem solving, distress, and sexual difficulties among cancer patients*. Paper presented at the 8th International Congress on Anti-Cancer Treatment, Paris.

Nezu, A. M., Nezu, C. M., & Blissett, S. E. (1988). Sense of humor as a moderator of the relation between stress-ful events and psychological distress: A prospective analysis. *Journal of Personality and Social Psychology, 54,* 520–525.

Nezu, A. M., Nezu, C. M., Faddis, S., DelliCarpini, L. A., & Houts, P. S. (1995, November). *Social problem solving as a moderator of cancer-related stress.* Paper presented at the annual meeting of the Association for the Advancement of Behavior Therapy, Washington, DC.

Nezu, A. M., Nezu, C. M., Friedman, S. H., Faddis, S., & Houts, P. S. (1997, November). *Problem-solving therapy for distressed cancer patients.* Paper presented at the annual meeting of the Association for the Advancement of Behavior Therapy, Miami, FL.

Nezu, A. M., Nezu, C. M., Friedman, S. H., & Haynes, S. N. (1997). Case formulation in behavior therapy. In T. D. Eells (Ed.), *Handbook of psychotherapy case formulation* (pp. 368–401). New York: Guilford Press.

Nezu, A. M., Nezu, C. M., Friedman, S. H., Houts, P. S., & Faddis, S. (1997). Project Genesis: Application of problem-solving therapy to psychosocial oncology. *The Behavior Therapist, 20,* 155–158.

Nezu, A. M., Nezu, C. M., Houts, P. S., Friedman, S. H., & Faddis, S. (in press). Relevance of problem-solving therapy to psychosocial oncology. *Journal of Psychosocial Oncology.*

Nezu, A. M., Nezu, C. M., & Perri, M. G. (1989). *Problem-solving therapy for depression: Theory, research, and clinical guidelines.* New York: Wiley.

Nezu, A. M., Nezu, C. M., Saraydarian, L., Kalmar, K., & Ronan, G. F. (1986). Social problem solving as a moderating variable between negative life stress and depression. *Cognitive Therapy and Research, 10,* 489–498.

Nezu, A. M., & Perri, M. G. (1989). Problem-solving therapy for unipolar depression: An initial dismantling investigation. *Journal of Consulting and Clinical Psychology, 57,* 408–413.

Nezu, A. M., Perri, M. G., & Nezu, C. M. (1987, August). *Validation of a problem solving/stress model of depression.* Paper presented at the 95th Annual Convention of the American Psychological Association, New York.

Nezu, A. M., Perri, M. G., Nezu, C. M., & Mahoney, D. (1987, November). *Social problem solving as a moderator of stressful events among clinically depressed individuals.* Paper presented at the annual meeting of the Association for the Advancement of Behavior Therapy, Boston.

Nezu, A. M., & Ronan, G. F. (1985). Life stress, current problems, problem solving, and depressive symptoms: An integrative model. *Journal of Consulting and Clinical Psychology, 53,* 693–697.

Nezu, A. M., & Ronan, G. F. (1987). Social problem solving and depression: Deficits in generating alternatives and decision making. *The Southern Psychologist, 3,* 29–34.

Nezu, A. M., & Ronan, G. F. (1988). Problem solving as a moderator of stress-related depressive symptoms: A prospective analysis. *Journal of Counseling Psychology, 35,* 134–138.

Nezu, C. M., & Nezu, A. M. (1995). Clinical decision making in everyday practice: The science in the art.

Cognitive and Behavioral Practice, 2, 5–25.

Nezu, C. M., Nezu, A. M., & Arean, P. A. (1991). Assertiveness and problem-solving therapy for mild mentally retarded persons with dual diagnoses. *Research in Developmental Disabilities, 12,* 371–386.

Nezu, C. M., Nezu, A. M., Friedman, S. H., Houts, P. S., DelliCarpini, L. A., Nemeth, C. B., & Faddis, S. (in press). Cancer and psychological distress: The role of problem solving. *Journal of Psychosocial Oncology.*

Nezu, C. M., Nezu, A. M., & Houts, P. S. (1993). The multiple applications of problem-solving principles in clinical practice. In K. T. Keuhlwein & H. Rosen (Eds.), *Cognitive therapy in action: Evolving innovative practice* (pp. 353–378). San Francisco: Jossey-Bass.

Oberst M. T., Thomas, S. E., Gass, M. A., & Ward, S. E. (1989). Caregiving demands and appraisal of stress among family caregivers. *Cancer Nursing, 12,* 209–215.

Parnes, S. J. (1967). *Creative problem-solving handbook.* New York: Scribner.

Perri, M. G., Nezu, A. M., & Viegener, B. J. (1992). *Improving the long-term management of obesity: Theory, research, and clinical guidelines.* New York: Wiley.

Pettingale, K. W., Morris, T., Greer, S., & Haybittle, J. L. (1985). Mental attitudes toward cancer: An additional prognostic factor. *The Lancet, 1,* 750.

Pfiffner, L. J., Jouriles, E. N., Brown, M. M., Etscheidt, M. A., & Kelly, J. A. (1990). Effects of problem-solving therapy on outcomes of parent training for single-parent families. *Child and Family Behavior Therapy, 12,* 1–11.

Phillips, S. D., Pazienza, N. J., & Ferrin, H. H. (1984). Decision making styles and problem solving appraisal. *Journal of Counseling Psychology, 31,* 497–502.

Platt, J. J., Husband, S. D., Hermalin, J., Cater, J., & Metzger, D. (1993). A cognitive problem-solving employment readiness intervention for methadone clients. *Journal of Cognitive Psychotherapy: An International Quarterly, 7,* 21–33.

Platt, J. J., & Spivack, G. (1974). Means of solving real-life problems: I. Psychiatric patients versus controls, and cross-cultural comparisons of normal females. *Journal of Community Psychology, 2,* 45–48.

Rabkin, J. G., & Klein, D. F. (1987). The clinical measurement of depressive disorders. In A. J. Marsella, R. M. A. Hirschfeld, & M. M. Katz (Eds.), *The measurement of depression* (pp. 30–83). New York: Guilford Press.

Rehm, L. P. (1981). A self-control therapy program for treatment of depression. In J. F. Clarkin & H. I. Glazer (Eds.), *Depression: Behavioral and directive intervention strategies* (pp. 68–110). New York: Guilford Press.

Richardson, J. L., Shelton, D. R., Krailo, M., & Levine, A. M. (1990). The effect of compliance with treatment on survival among patients with hematologic malignancies. *Journal of Clinical Oncology, 8,* 356–364.

Rogers, C. R. (1957). The necessary and sufficient conditions of therapeutic personality change. *Journal of Consulting and Clinical Psychology, 21,* 95–103.

Rothenberg, J. L., Nezu, A. M., Nezu, C. M., & Swain, R. (1994, November). *Problem-solving skills as a moderator of distress in caregivers of Alzheimer's disease.* Paper presented at the annual meeting of the Association for the Advancement of Behavior Therapy, San Diego, CA.

Rotter, J. B. (1966). Generalized expectancies for internal versus external control of reinforcement. *Psychological Monographs, 80*, 1–28.

Rowland, J. H. (1990a). Intrapersonal resources: Coping. In J. C. Holland & J. H. Rowland (Eds.), *Handbook of psychooncology* (pp. 44–57). New York: Oxford University Press.

Rowland, J. H. (1990b). Interpersonal resources: Social support. In J. C. Holland & J. H. Rowland (Eds.), *Handbook of psychooncology* (pp. 58–71). New York: Oxford University Press.

Sacco, W. P., & Graves, D. J. (1984). Childhood depression, interpersonal problem solving, and self-ratings of performance. *Journal of Clinical Child Psychology, 13*, 10–15.

Salkovskis, P. M., Atha, C., & Storer, D. (1990). Cognitive–behavioural problem solving in the treatment of patients who repeatedly attempt suicide: A controlled trial. *British Journal of Psychiatry, 157*, 871–876.

Sarason, I. G., Johnson, J. H., & Siegel, J. M. (1978). Assessing the impact of life changes: Development of the Life Experiences Survey. *Journal of Consulting and Clinical Psychology, 46*, 932–946.

Schag, C. A. C., & Heinrich, R. L. (1989). *The Cancer Rehabilitation Evaluation System (CARES): Manual.* Los Angeles: CARES Consultants.

Schag, C. A. C., Heinrich, R. L., Aadland, R. L., & Ganz, P. A. (1990). Assessing problems of cancer patients: Psychometric properties of the Cancer Inventory of Problem Situations. *Health Psychology, 9*, 83–102.

Schag, C. C., Heinrich, R. L., & Ganz, P. A. (1983). The Cancer Inventory of Problem Situations: An instrument for assessing cancer patients' rehabilitation needs. *Journal of Psychosocial Oncology, 1*, 11–24.

Schinka, J. A. (1986). *Personal problems checklist.* Odessa, FL: Psychological Assessment Resources.

Schipper, H., Clinch, J., McMurray, A., & Levitt, M. (1984). Measuring the quality of life of cancer patients: The Functional Living Index—Cancer: Development and validation. *Journal of Clinical Oncology, 2*, 472–483.

Schotte, D. E., & Clum, G. A. (1982). Suicide ideation in a college population. *Journal of Consulting and Clinical Psychology, 50*, 690–696.

Schotte, D. E., & Clum, G. A. (1987). Problem-solving skills in suicidal psychiatric patients. *Journal of Consulting and Clinical Psychology, 58*, 49–54.

Sherry, P., Keitel, M., & Tracey, T. J. (1984, August). *The relationship between person–environment fit, coping, and strain.* Paper presented at the 92nd Annual Convention of the American Psychological Association, Toronto, Ontario, Canada.

Spiegel, D., Bloom, J. R., Kraemer, H. C., & Gottheil, E. (1989). Effects of psychosocial treatment on survival patients with metastatic breast cancer. *The Lancet, 2*, 888–891.

Spielberger, C. D., Gorsuch, R. L., & Lushene, R. E. (1979). *Manual for the State–Trait Anxiety Inventory.* Palo Alto, CA: Consulting Psychologists Press.

Spitzer, W. O., Dobson, A. J., Hall, J., Chesterman, E., Levi, J., Shepherd,

R., Battista, R. N., & Catchlove, B. R. (1981). Measuring the quality of life of cancer patients: A concise QL-Index for use by physicians. *Journal of Chronic Diseases, 34*, 585–597.

Telch, C. F., & Telch, M. J. (1986). Group coping skills instruction and supportive group therapy for cancer patients: A comparison of strategies. *Journal of Consulting and Clinical Psychology, 54*, 802–808.

Temoshok, L. (1985). Biopsychosocial studies on cutaneous malignant melanoma: Psychosocial factors associated with prognostic indicators, progression, psychophysiology and tumor–host response. *Social Science in Medicine, 20*, 833–840.

Thompson, S. C., & Collins, M. A. (1995). Applications of perceived control to cancer: An overview of theory and measurement. *Journal of Psychosocial Oncology, 13*, 11–26.

Thompson, S. C., & Pitts, J. (1993). Factors relating to a person's ability to find meaning after a diagnosis of cancer. *Journal of Psychosocial Oncology, 11*, 1–21.

Tross, S., & Holland, J. C. (1990). Psychological sequelae in cancer survivors. In J. C. Holland & J. H. Rowland (Eds.), *Handbook of psychooncology* (pp. 101–116). New York: Oxford University Press.

Truax, C. B., & Carkhuff, R. R. (1967). *Toward effective counseling and psychotherapy*. Chicago: Aldine.

Twycross, R. G., & Lack, S. A. (1983). *Symptom control in far advanced cancer: Pain relief*. London: Pitman.

Vinokur, A. D., Threatt, B. A., Vinokur-Kaplan, D., & Satariano, W. A. (1990). The process of recovery from breast cancer for younger and older patients. *Cancer, 65*, 1242–1254.

Wan, G. J., Counte, M. A., & Cella, D. F. (1997). The influence of personal expectations on cancer patients' reports of health-related quality of life. *Psycho-oncology, 6*, 1–11.

Ware, J. E., & Sherbourne, C. D. (1992). The MOS 36-Item Short Form Health Survey (SF-36): I. Conceptual framework and item selection. *Medical Care, 30*, 473–483.

Watson, M., Greer, S., Prieyn, J., & Van Den Bourne, B. (1990). Locus of control and adjustment to cancer. *Psychological Reports, 66*, 39–48.

Watson, M., & Ramirez, A. (1991). Psychological factors in cancer prognosis. In C. L. Cooper & M. Watson (Eds.), *Cancer and stress: Psychological, biological and coping studies* (pp. 47–71). Chicheser, England: Wiley.

Weisman, A. D., & Worden, J. W. (1976–1977). The existential plight in cancer: Significance of the first 100 days. *International Journal of Psychiatric Medicine, 7*, 1–15.

Weisman, A. D., Worden, J. W., & Sobel, H. J. (1980). *Psychosocial screening and intervention with cancer patients* (Tech. Rep. No. CA-19797). Bethesda, MD: National Cancer Institute.

Whitlock, F. A. (1978). Suicide, cancer and depression. *British Journal of Psychiatry, 132*, 269–274.

Yesavitch, J., Brink, T., Rose, T., Lum, O., Huang, O., Adey, V., & Leier, V. (1983). Development and validation of a geriatric screening scale: A preliminary report. *Journal of Psychiatric Research, 17*, 37–49.

Young, J., & Swift, W. (1988). Schema-focused cognitive therapy for personality disorders: Part I. *International Cognitive Therapy Newsletter, 4*, 13–14.

Zabora, J. R., Smith-Wilson, R., Fetting, J. H., & Enterline, J. P. (1990). An efficient method for psychosocial screening of cancer patients. *Psychosomatics, 31,* 192–196.

Zemore, R., & Dell, L. W. (1983). Interpersonal problem-solving skills and depression proneness. *Personality and Social Psychology Bulletin, 9,* 231–235.

Index

About the Authors

Arthur M. Nezu, PhD, is currently Professor and Chair of the Department of Clinical and Health Psychology at Allegheny University of the Health Sciences in Philadelphia, where he also serves as Senior Associate Dean for Research, Associate Director of the Center for Mind/Body Studies, and Professor of Medicine (Medical Oncology) and Public Health. He is a Fellow of the American Psychological Association, the American Psychological Society, the American Association of Applied and Prevention Psychology, and the Society for Behavioral Medicine. He serves on the editorial boards of numerous journals, including the *Journal of Consulting and Clinical Psychology,* and is currently editor of *the Behavior Therapist.* He has over 100 publications on a variety of health and mental health topics, and his writings have been translated into Japanese, Italian, French, Danish, and Spanish. He is President-Elect of the Association for Advancement of Behavior Therapy. His research in psycho-oncology has been supported by the National Cancer Institute, including Project Genesis.

Christine Maguth Nezu, PhD, is currently Associate Professor of Clinical and Health Psychology and Medicine (Medical Oncology), as well as the Director of the Center for Mind/Body Studies at Allegheny University of the Health Sciences, where until recently she also served as Associate Provost for Research and Scientific Integrity Officer. She has coauthored more than 50 research publications concerning behavioral medicine, aggressive and violent behavior, clinical decision making, psychopathology, and developmental disabilities. She served as co-principal investigator for several federally-funded research projects, including Project Genesis, that support the efficacy of problem-solving therapy for the treatment of psychological and emotional distress in cancer